SAFE NATURAL REMEDIES
FOR BABIES AND CHILDREN

BY THE SAME AUTHOR:

The Encyclopaedia of Flower Remedies
(with Clare Harvey; Thorsons)

Dolphins and Their Power to Heal
(with Karena Callen; Bloomsbury)

SAFE NATURAL REMEDIES
FOR BABIES AND CHILDREN

Amanda Cochrane

Thorsons
An Imprint of HarperCollinsPublishers

For Hamish and Katharine

Thorsons
An Imprint of HarperCollinsPublishers
77–85 Fulham Palace Road,
Hammersmith, London W6 8JB

1160 Battery Street,
San Francisco, California 94111–1213

Published by Thorsons 1997

3 5 7 9 10 8 6 4

© Amanda Cochrane 1997

Amanda Cochrane asserts the moral right to
be identified as the author of this work

A catalogue record for this book
is available from the British Library

ISBN 0 7225 3369 1

Printed and bound in Great Britain by
Clays Ltd, St Ives plc

All rights reserved. No part of this publication may be
reproduced, stored in a retrieval system, or transmitted,
in any form or by any means, electronic, mechanical,
photocopying, recording or otherwise, without the prior
permission of the publishers.

Contents

Acknowledgements vi
Foreword vii
Introduction viii

PART I THE NATURAL THERAPIES 1

Aromatherapy 2
Biochemic Tissue Salts 8
Chinese Medicine 10
Diet and Nutritional Therapy 16
Flower Remedies 24
Herbal Medicine 27
Homoeopathy 34
Hydrotherapy 39
Massage 42
Naturopathy 47
Osteopathy 49
Reflexology 51
Relaxation, Rest and Sleep 55
The Natural Medicine Chest 57

PART II A–Z OF CHILDHOOD AILMENTS 59

Addresses 280
References and Further Reading 288

Acknowledgements

Thank you to all those who have given generously of their expertise and knowledge.

Consultants:

MEDICAL – Dr Nuala Galazka, a family GP, for providing the 'Doctor's Prescriptions' and ensuring that the information in this book is medically safe and sound.

AROMATHERAPY – Colette Prideaux-Brune, a mother and highly respected aromatherapist with much experience in treating babies and children, for advising on the best aromatherapy oils to use at home.

CHINESE MEDICINE – Katherine Jackson, a respected practitioner of Chinese medicine and herbalism, for information on Chinese herbal remedies and acupressure points to use for different ailments.

FLOWER REMEDIES – Clare Harvey, the country's leading flower remedy practitioner, for recommendations of appropriate flower essences for different conditions.

HERBALISM – Marion Bielby, a mother of four and herbal practitioner with considerable experience of treating children with herbs and herbal remedies, for endorsing the remedies recommended in this book and for providing recipes for home use.

HOMOEOPATHY – Annette Middleton, a fully qualified homoeopath, for her advice and endorsement of the homoeopathic recommendations for different ailments.

NATUROPATHY – Dr Ian Drysdale, Director of the British College of Naturopathy and Osteopathy, for his naturopathic advice and recommendations.

OSTEOPATHY – Stuart Korth, Director of the Osteopathic Centre for Children, for his overview of the relevance of osteopathy in the treatment of children's ailments.

Foreword

The health and safety of our children is one of the few fundamentals of life. Over the decades we have been encouraged to use modern medicine as the first point of call when a child is ill, when in fact many of the gentler complementary treatments may offer a more effective cure.

As a mother, I know how deeply agonizing it is when our child is ill. We instinctively seek out the speediest and most effective remedy. Above all, though, we want to be sure that the treatments we are given to use are safe. Unfortunately, conventional drug compounds are frequently accompanied by side-effects and contra-indications. They also tend to treat only the visible symptoms instead of tackling the underlying causes of the problem. By contrast, many traditional remedies such as homoeopathy, herbalism and osteopathy can be so very effective because they address the human body as a whole (hence the concept of 'holistic' medicine) and treat the root cause of the disorder, helping to ensure that it does not return.

I have had the pleasure of knowing the author of this book for many years, both as a friend and colleague. However, as a health writer and broadcaster I was especially pleased to read the sections Amanda has compiled on diet and nutritional therapy and also on naturopathy, as both these disciplines have a great deal to offer children and yet are overlooked in the many childcare manuals that line my bookshelves.

Safe Natural Remedies for Babies and Children is a wonderful reference source for all the family. It gives good advice on a wide range of ailments from birth to beyond. I have even used some of the suggestions for my 90-year-old grandmother, proving that the fundamentals of good health are indeed ageless. Fitness and vitality are two of the most precious gifts that we as parents can pass on to our offspring. I'm sure that this book will help to ensure the very best of health for you and your family, both now and in the years ahead.

Liz Earle
London, 1997

Introduction

No matter how well you care for your child, all babies and young children are susceptible to a wide range of ailments. For some parents the enjoyment of the precious early months and years can be marred by what seems like an endless stream of minor health problems. It is always worrying when your child falls ill. Even the happiest and most carefree babies and children are often fractious, clingy and miserable when they feel unwell.

This is where natural remedies come to the rescue. They are safe, gentle, effective and can help to bring relief from most common childhood ailments while encouraging a speedy recovery. These natural remedies not only soothe symptoms, they actually stimulate the body's own natural healing powers to restore vitality and generally enhance resistance to other illnesses.

There are a wide variety of natural remedies which can be safely used for babies and children. They take the form of essential oils (aromatherapy), herbal tinctures and tisanes (herbalism), homoeopathic remedies (homoeopathy), therapeutic baths (naturopathy), medicinal foods (diet and nutritional therapy) and massage and the stimulation of certain pressure points on the body (acupressure and reflexology).

Being sensitive, babies and children respond particularly well to these subtle forms of treatment. The beauty of all the natural remedies described given in this book is that they are completely safe even for tiny babies, and free from any possible side-effects.

In many instances natural remedies work most effectively when used in combination. For instance, a qualified practitioner of Chinese medicine can recommend key acupressure points to enhance the therapeutic potential of herbal preparations; massage can be used in conjunction with essential oils to potentiate its soothing or energizing effects; the benefits of homoeopathic remedies may be enhanced by following certain dietary advice.

You may also find that your child accepts or responds to one type of treatment or remedy better than to others. Children tend to know what is best for them, so follow their instincts as well as your own.

Prevention Is Better than Cure

Natural remedies play a particularly valuable role in preventing as well as relieving all kinds of illnesses. Essential oils used in aromatherapy, for example, are all naturally antiseptic and, when used on a regular basis, can offer protection from various infections, especially coughs and colds. Nourishing foods offer some of the best protection against all kinds of ills; certain nutrients in particular can help in relieving various psychological problems such as hyperactivity and irritability as well as physical complaints. Essential oils, herbal tisanes and homoeopathic remedies are undoubtedly more effective when your child is well-nourished and has a healthy lifestyle.

When given at the first sign of sickness or discomfort, natural remedies can also help to nip potential health problems in the bud. While they are not intended to replace conventional medical treatment, they may preclude the need for any stronger forms of medication. Giving homoeopathic Chamomilla drops to a teething baby, for example, can be as soothing as a dose of pain-relief syrup.

Natural remedies also come into their own when doctors are reluctant to prescribe medication unless absolutely necessary. Most GPs are increasingly hesitant about giving antibiotics for colds and other infections, as overuse of these drugs in the past has led to the development of drug-resistant strains of bacteria. This can leave you feeling slightly at a loss for what to give a child who is suffering with a sore throat, stuffy head and streaming nose. Luckily there are many natural remedies which can help to soothe symptoms such as these and strengthen the body's own immune defences, to enable your child to shake off infections.

At times when your child may need conventional medication, natural remedies can safely be used alongside most orthodox prescriptions and will actually help your child to make a speedier recovery.

Helping Your Child Back to Health

Caring for a child who is unwell is not only a question of choosing the correct remedy. Babies and children become much more needy when ill and desire plenty of tender loving care. Cuddles and comfort are all part and parcel of helping your child to feel better again.

The desire to get better is very strong in most children and they should be encouraged to take part in their own healing process whenever they can. It is a good idea to explain what you are doing to make them feel better again: involve them as much as possible.

Suggestion and creative imagery can be extremely therapeutic, hence the power of the placebo. Many healers find a child's imagination can be brought into play very successfully in stimulating recovery. Try asking your child to find a 'magic' stone, feather, leaf or shell to help him feel well again; let him take it to bed. Nor should the power of simply 'kissing it better' be underestimated.

Young children can also learn for themselves how to work certain acupressure points or reflex zones on the hands and feet to soothe a stomach ache or relieve an attack of hay fever, for example.

Looking after yourself when caring for a sick child is also important. When children are ill it is difficult to keep from being anxious, worried, irritable and weary from lack of sleep. Children are affected by the moods of those caring for them and they need you to be calm, relaxed and strong when they are unwell. Some of the remedies in this book may therefore be helpful for you too, so you can give your child plenty of time and attention without becoming too tired.

How to Use this Book

Part One introduces a wide range of natural therapies and remedies, from Aromatherapy through Relaxation techniques. You will discover the principles of each natural therapy, the way its remedies work and the kind of ailments it can help to treat and prevent.

Part Two is the A–Z of Childhood Ailments. It tells you a little about each health problem and its typical symptoms. The most effective natural remedies for treating each illness are highlighted, along with various other helpful therapies you might try. Whenever relevant there is also a section on practical advice and a typical 'doctor's prescription' – that is, the treatment offered by orthodox medicine.

Please remember that these natural remedies are not designed to take the place of proper medical care. Contact your doctor at once if ever your child:

* has a temperature of 39°C/102.2°F or higher
* cannot be woken
* has a fit or convulsion
* is unusually 'floppy'
* seems to be in severe pain

- * inhales a foreign body into the lungs
- * has persistent sickness or diarrhoea
- * passes blood-stained stools
- * has breathing difficulties or turns blue
- * shows signs of meningitis (headache, stiff neck, high temperature, sensitive eyes).

Please note that throughout this book we have used 'he' to mean any child, to avoid the somewhat unwieldy 'he or she'.

Part One

The Natural Therapies

Aromatherapy

Aromatherapy is the practice of using scented plant oils known as 'essential oils' to enhance health and restore a feeling of well-being. These fragrant oils are blessed with many therapeutic properties which help to prevent health problems and provide gentle relief for all kinds of symptoms.

The medicinal use of aromatic substances goes back to the ancient Chinese, Indian, Hebrew and Arab civilizations. Aromatherapy flourished with the ancient Egyptians, Greeks and Romans. By the turn of the 18th century, essential oils were widely used in medicinal preparations.

The term aromatherapy was first used by the French scientist René Gattefossé in the 1920s. During a laboratory experiment he burned his hand badly; by chance, a bowl of Lavender oil was nearby. He plunged his burnt hand into this and, to his surprise, the pain subsided and his skin healed rapidly without scarring.

The Benefits of Aromatherapy

Essential oils are extracted from the flowers, leaves, stems, roots or bark of various aromatic plants. Rose essence, for example, comes from the rose petals, Lemon essence from lemon rind and Ginger essence from ginger root. Each essential oil has its own distinctive aroma and 'profile' of therapeutic properties. While essential oils such as Rose and Jasmine are valued as perfumes, when choosing the best ones for babies and children the medicinal qualities of an oil are of primary importance.

Most essential oils are naturally antiseptic and will inhibit bacterial growth. Some are stronger than others. The more potent ones, such as Tea Tree and Eucalyptus, appear to strengthen the body's own immune defences, helping to ward off and overcome all kinds of minor infections. Others, including Chamomile and Lavender, will help to reduce inflammation, pain and swelling. Still others, such as Geranium and, again, Lavender, encourage cell regeneration and are therefore excellent for use on bumps and bruises.

Soothing Scents

Essential oils can have a positive influence on your child's emotional well-being, too. Babies and children are highly sensitive to smell. A few days after birth a newborn baby already associates mother's subtle skin scent with comfort, warmth, food and security. If you dab a few drops of an essential oil (such as Rose or Lavender) behind your ears, your baby will come to associate this aroma with you. Then if the baby finds it difficult to settle if you are not there, a few drops of your personal essence on the cot bumper or a teddy may soothe him.

Some essential oils contain chemicals which are mildly sedative and can calm over-excited children. Others have a gentle tonic effect and act as pick-me-ups, helping to revive natural vitality.

Preference for aromas is highly individual. What appeals to one child another may find repellent! Most young children seem to prefer the fresh, uplifting citrus aromas such as Lemon, Mandarin and Sweet Orange. Experiment until you find the one your child seems to like best.

Using Essential Oils

ON THE SKIN

Smoothing an oil containing a few drops of essential oils into the skin combines the benefits of massage and aromatherapy. As essential oils are so concentrated, they must always be blended with a carrier oil before being used in this way. Never drop them directly onto a baby or young child's skin, as they can sting and cause irritation.

To dilute an essential oil, add 1–3 drops of the oil to 5 ml of a vegetable oil such as Almond, Avocado, Grapeseed or Wheatgerm.

If making a larger quantity, store the unused oil in a tinted bottle and keep in a cool place to preserve its therapeutic benefits.

IN THE BATH

By using essential oils in the bath your child will benefit from inhaling the vapours and absorbing them through the skin. When adding essential oils to the bath, always dilute them first in a teaspoon of base oil, milk or honey. As young children tend to suck sponges and drink the bath water, this will safeguard against ingesting neat essential oils from the surface. Add the oils to the bath while the hot water is running and swirl the bath water around to disperse the drops. To enjoy the full benefits of an aromatherapy bath your child should stay in the water for at least 10 minutes.

INHALATION OR VAPORIZATION

This is an ideal way of freshening your child's bedroom and inhibiting the spread of infection through the family.

There are various ways to vaporize essential oils. You can add a few drops to a bowl of steaming hot water so the aroma fills the room. There are electric vaporizers which can be used if your child is mobile and you are worried about leaving a bowl of hot water where they might reach it. Other vaporizers plug directly into a socket and are good for using at night-time in a baby's bedroom.

Another option is to put a few drops of essential oil onto a ball of dampened cotton wool and placing it on the radiator, or adding a few drops to an atomizer such as a plant spray (5 drops to 8 fl oz/ 250 ml of water) and spraying around the room.

Essential Oils for Babies and Children

There are many different essential oils, not all of which are suitable or completely safe for babies and children. For newborns only a handful of essential oils are recommended. You can use additional essences as your child gets older, adding to this repertoire as the months and years go by.

For young babies and children choose just one of the essences recommended below. For children over 6 years old you can make simple blends of two different essential oils.

AGE	ESSENCES YOU CAN USE
Newborn to 2 months	Chamomile, Lavender, Fennel, Dill
2 to 6 months	as above, plus Sweet Orange
6 to 12 months	as above, plus Eucalyptus and Tea Tree
1 to 5 years	as above, plus Peppermint and Geranium
5 to 7 years	as above, plus Thyme, Hyssop, Patchouli, Black Pepper, Marjoram, Rosemary, Sandalwood, Niaouli, Lemon and Ginger
over 7 years	as above, plus Frankincense, Melissa, Basil, Rose, Benzoin and Bergamot

DOSAGES

Aromatherapy preparations for very young babies should be well diluted. As your child gets older you can add a few more drops to the carrier oil.

AGE	BATH	DROPS PER 30 ML BASE OIL
Newborn to 2 months	1–2 drops	1–2 drops
2 to 6 months	1–2 drops	2–3 drops
6 to 12 months	2–3 drops	3–4 drops
1 to 5 years	2–3 drops	4–6 drops
5 to 7 years	3–4 drops	6–10 drops
7 to 12 years	4–5 drops	8–12 drops

Choosing Essential Oils

Essential oils intended for therapeutic use should be pure and natural, extracted from organically grown plants whenever possible.

High-grade essential oils tend to be more expensive than those doctored with synthetic additives to make them smell attractive. However, many good quality essential oils are reasonably priced and can be recommended for everyday use (*see page 280 for recommended suppliers*).

Vegetable Carrier Oils

* Almond oil: rich in vitamin E; good for dry skin, helps to soothe inflammation and relieve itching
* Avocado oil: contains vitamin A; encourages skin healing and helps to treat dry skin conditions such as eczema and psoriasis
* Grapeseed oil: contains vitamins E and F; very mild and recommended for those with allergic tendencies

- Olive oil: rich and very emollient; helps to relieve itching and can be used on insect bites, burns, bruises and sprains
- Rosehip oil: encourages regeneration of skin; good for burns including sunburn, cuts, scratches, eczema and psoriasis
- Sunflower oil: contains vitamins A, D and E; good for bruises
- Wheatgerm oil: rich in vitamin E; better for children over 6 years old. Helps to treat dry skin conditions.

Safety Tips

- Essential oils are highly volatile and flammable, so must always be kept away from fire or flames of any kind.
- Always store essential oils in a cool, dark place out of your children's reach. The safest bottles have a dropper insert which will prevent a child from accidentally swallowing any essence should he get hold of it. Pipette bottles are not safe to use with children around.
- Do not use a candle burner in children's bedrooms. Instead use an electric vaporizer or place drops on your child's pillow case or pyjamas.
- Never give your child essential oils to swallow.
- Neat essential oils should not be applied directly to the skin unless specified – for example, Lavender can be dabbed onto minor burns.
- Do not attempt to treat a child who is seriously ill without first contacting your doctor.

Biochemic Tissue Salts

Biochemic tissue salts are extremely gentle remedies; they are particularly suitable for infants. They are prepared in the same way as homoeopathic medicines (*see page 34*), containing highly dilute quantities of mineral salts in a base of lactose (milk sugar). However, whereas homoeopathy treats like with like, tissue salts work by seeking to redress imbalances in the body. They come in tablet form and are absorbed quickly by the body. They are thought to bring quick relief for a wide range of ailments.

How Tissue Salts Work

The concept of biochemic tissue salts was developed in the 1870s by a German homoeopathic physician, Dr Wilhelm Schuessler. As a result of his research, Schuessler discovered 12 mineral salts occurring naturally in the body. These salts, he suggested, play an important role in enabling the body cells to function properly. His discovery has been verified by recent research which shows that there are indeed at least 12 tissue salts in the body.

Schuessler believed that everyday health problems such as coughs and colds are associated with an imbalance of these mineral tissue salts. By taking the correct formulation of mineral salts you are helping to re-balance cell metabolism and enable the body to shake off the illness.

Prescribing for your baby or child is simple. Note the symptoms and then select the salt or combination of salts recommended for them. Each salt is known by a number and an abbreviated name. A combination remedy is known by a letter.

The small, moulded, lactose-based tablets dissolve quickly in the mouth. They can be taken every half hour if the symptoms are sudden and short-lived; every two hours if they are long lasting. Tissue salts have no unpleasant side-effects and there is no risk of over-dosing as the quantities are so minute.

BIOCHEMIC REMEDIES SUITABLE FOR BABIES AND CHILDREN	
Calc phos (calcium phosphate)	poor circulation, indigestion, lowered vitality, weak teeth, iron-deficiency anaemia
Ferr phos (iron phosphate)	inflammation of the skin, feverishness, chestiness, sore throat, coughs, colds, chills
Kali mur (potassium chloride)	respiratory disorders such as asthma and bronchitis; catarrh, colds, wheezing, sore throat, tonsillitis, sluggish digestion
Kali sulph (potassium sulphate)	a nerve soother useful for tension, headaches, indigestion, loss of sleep and irritability due to worry or excitement
Kali phos	minor skin eruptions with scaling; discharge from the nose or throat, catarrh; problems affecting the nails, hair and scalp
Mag phos (magnesium phosphate)	relief of darting pains, cramp and hiccups, colic and wind
Nat mur (sodium chloride)	'watery' colds (accompanied by tears and a runny nose); loss of smell or taste
Nat sulph (sodium sulphate)	nausea, queasiness, digestive problems, colic, influenza symptoms and headaches

COMBINATION REMEDIES	
Combination D	minor skin ailments
Combination E	flatulence, indigestion
Combination H	hayfever
Combination J	coughs, colds and chestiness
Combination Q	catarrh, sinus disorders
Combination R	infants' teething problems

Chinese Medicine

Chinese medicine is based on principles that most people living in the West are unfamiliar with. Dating back at least 4,000 years, traditional Chinese medicine sees people (and all living creatures) as being infused with a subtle energy known as *qi* or *chi*. This is a sort of 'life force' which gives us vitality and is said to be particularly abundant in babies and young children. In good health, *qi* is balanced and flows freely.

Qi moves along a network of channels called meridians which spread like an intricate web through the body. There are 12 pairs of meridians, and each pair governs a particular organ such as the kidneys, or a bodily function such as circulation. Health problems arise when the movement of *qi* along any meridian is upset. The *qi* can thus become blocked and depleted, or may accumulate and become excessive.

Chinese medicine provides various ways of restoring the smooth flow of *qi* to revive vitality and relieve symptoms. More importantly, it places particular emphasis on keeping *qi* in balance and so preventing health problems from arising in the first place. If steps are taken throughout childhood to maintain this balance, your child may be less vulnerable to health problems later in life.

Acupressure

The Chinese have been using acupressure for centuries to preserve and restore the balance of *qi*.

This healing art uses finger pressure on key acupuncture points over the body. These points can be visualized as tiny pinpricks of light dotted along the meridians. They are like windows through which you can literally 'tap' into the body's *qi*. Acupressure is thought to be the forerunner of acupuncture, which uses needles to stimulate these points. It is still widely used at home by many Chinese families for soothing infant colic, treating headaches, and relieving insomnia and other upsets.

Although acupressure seems to be a very subtle form of treatment, scientific studies suggest it does have a therapeutic effect. Research at the Department of Anaesthetics at Belfast University has shown clearly that acupressure or an acupressure band worn on a point called Pericardium 6 does indeed relieve the nausea caused by travel sickness, as well as that caused by pregnancy, general anaesthesia and some drugs.

Acupressure is now being evaluated in the same way as any other promising new treatment. The beauty of acupressure is that it is painless, has no side-effects and is simple to perform.

HOW TO GIVE AN ACUPRESSURE TREATMENT

Practitioners use a firm thumb or fingertip massage on key acupuncture points. You can do the same for your baby or child. Choose a moment when he is feeling calm and relaxed, perhaps while you are reading a bedtime story together. Find the pressure points you need to work, as highlighted for particular ailments. Press firmly with the pad of your first finger or thumb, then release, press and release over and over again (do not dig your nail into the skin). For babies begin by working each point for about half a minute; applying pressure for longer as your child becomes used to this treatment.

Points where there is an energy block are often tender. However, this treatment should never be painful and if your child finds it uncomfortable or unpleasant, don't persist as you risk putting him off for ever.

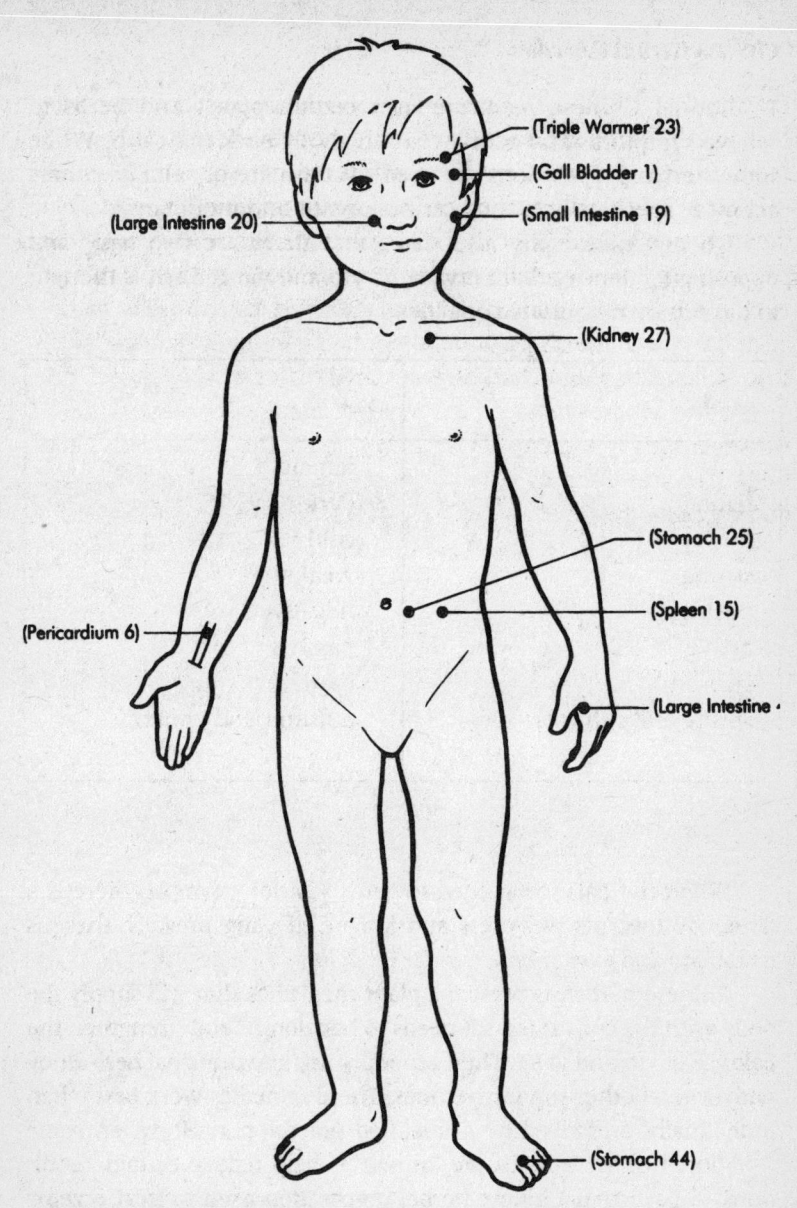

FIGURE 1: ACUPRESSURE POINTS

Chinese Herbal Remedies

Traditional Chinese medicine uses certain plants and herbs to relieve symptoms and gently coax the body back to health. While some herbal preparations are used to stimulate or calm *qi*, others act more specifically to tone certain organs and meridians.

Oriental philosophy also states that there are two basic and opposing tendencies that pervade *qi*: yin and yang. Each is thought to have its own associated qualities:

YANG	YIN
male	female
light	dark
hot	cold
strong	weak
positive	negative
active	passive
sun	earth
spring and summer	autumn and winter

When the balance is tilted towards yin, for example, there is a tendency towards weakness and fatigue. If yang prevails, there is irritability and excitation.

Chinese herbalists prescribe plant medicines that will supply the body with the constituents it needs to harmonize and strengthen the balance of yin and yang. They generally use one principal herb along with several other supportive ones. These remedies work best when individually prescribed by a qualified practitioner. However, some traditional Chinese herbs are known to help relieve certain conditions. A particular Chinese herbal preparation used to treat eczema was recently evaluated scientifically (the results were published in the medical journal *The Lancet*) and found to be as effective as the cortico-steroid drugs usually prescribed to combat this condition.

The Chinese herbal medicines recommended in this book are simple home remedies that have been used to treat particular health problems for centuries. Herbs, flowers, leaves or blossoms are prepared as ordinary *tisanes* – the plant is placed in a pan, boiling water is poured over and it is left to steep.

Hard substances such as roots and barks are prepared as *decoctions* (boiled continuously for a certain length of time). Herbal *tinctures* (ground or chopped herbs left to steep in alcohol) can also be used and may be preferable in some instances.

While safe and totally non-toxic, it is important to follow the dosage recommendations for any herbal remedy taken.

Important note: it is not advisable to give Chinese herbal remedies to babies under 6 months of age.

Dosages

INFUSIONS AND DECOCTIONS

Pour half a pint (300 ml) of boiling water over 1 teaspoon of the fresh herb. Leave to steep for 10 minutes.

Dilute the resulting tisane with the same quantity (half a pint/300 ml) of mineral water and give as sips when tepid.

TINCTURES	
Newborn to 6 months	Breastfeeding mothers can take 1 teaspoon of tincture in 1 cup (240 ml) of just boiled water, 3 times a day
6 months to 3 years	5 drops in a wineglass (180 ml) of cooled boiled water, twice a day
3 to 10 years	10 drops in a wineglass (180 ml) of cooled boiled water, twice a day

Diet and Nutritional Therapy

A wholesome diet plays a vital role in maintaining good health. Eating fresh natural foods which provide the entire spectrum of essential nutrients will help babies and children to be more resistant to all kinds of health problems. A well-nourished child can shake off an infection or illness with ease, and will make a speedy recovery if he does fall ill.

Children with a healthy diet also respond better to natural medicines. Eating the wrong foods may actually exacerbate or even lie at the root of problems such as eczema, hyperactivity and asthma.

The ideal diet is composed of a wide range of fresh, natural foods, including:

* fresh fruits and vegetables, especially green leafy varieties
* wholegrain cereals such as brown rice, wholewheat bread, wholemeal pasta, oat flakes, barley, rye and maize
* fish such as salmon and cod, and oily varieties such as sardines and mackerel
* poultry
* eggs
* meat – lamb, beef, pork
* dairy produce – milk, yoghurt and cheese (ideally, cow's milk should not be included in the diet until after 12 months of age)
* nuts – walnuts, hazelnuts, almonds (not peanuts) and seeds – sunflower, pumpkin and sesame, which can be ground and sprinkled onto yoghurt and cereals.

These foods should provide all the nutrients a growing child requires. Nowadays, however, ensuring your child has a healthy diet is not always easy. As parents we are bombarded with 'speciality' foods to tempt our children. These are generally high in refined carbohydrates, laden with sugar or salt, spiced up with flavourings and brightened with artificial colourings. These foods provide empty calories – energy without sufficient quantities of the nutrients needed to process it properly. Nutritional deficiencies are more likely to occur in children whose diet is based on such foods. Eating too many refined carbohydrates and sugars uses up the body's supplies of B vitamins and minerals such as zinc and magnesium.

A nationwide survey reveals that deficiencies of iron and zinc are quite prevalent in young children. The National Diet and Nutrition Survey commissioned by the Government and published in 1995 found that the intake of iron was considerably lower than the recommended nutrient intake in 21 per cent of 6- to 12-month-olds and 16 per cent of those aged between 18 months and 4 years. Around 10 per cent of children actually have iron-deficiency anaemia. The classic symptoms of anaemia include fatigue, tiredness, dizziness, a pale complexion, reduced growth and increased susceptibility to infections. Iron deficiency can also be a cause of behavioural problems and can adversely affect cognitive function, especially language skills and body balance.

Poor zinc status is also fairly common. Around 6 per cent of babies between 6 and 12 months old are zinc deficient, a statistic that rises to 14 per cent for those ages between 18 months and 4 years. A lack of zinc is linked to poor resistance to infections, sleeplessness in babies and young children, skin conditions such as eczema and many other health problems.

Recent research also suggests that the kind of diet we eat during the first six years of life will determine our food preferences for the rest of our lives. Creating an unnatural taste for sweet, salty or artificially flavoured foods at an early age makes it increasingly difficult to introduce healthy foods later on. This is another reason why it is best to begin good habits in babyhood with fresh, home-made meals. Even commercial baby foods often contain unnecessary fillers such as refined starch and sugar.

Healthy Hints

* Start the day with a home-made muesli made with fine oat flakes, grated apple, sultanas, chopped dates and a little milk. Alternatively, give your child slices of lightly buttered wholemeal toast or natural yoghurt sweetened with honey and/or fresh fruit.

* Offer sticks of raw vegetables and fruits to snack on between meals, rather than cakes and biscuits. Carrots, celery, apples, bananas, sliced grapes and pears are ideal, as are strawberries, raspberries, peaches and pineapple during the summer months.

* Dried fruits such as raisins, sultanas, apricots, peaches, pears, dates and figs make a good alternative to sweets.

* When children are older (over 3 years old) or when you feel they are ready you can add unsalted nuts such as almonds, Brazil nuts, walnuts and pecans to their diet. It is best to avoid peanuts, as some children can have an extreme allergic reaction to them.

Medicinal Foods

Some foods are traditionally regarded as having therapeutic properties. Many of these are rich sources of certain nutrients. Lemons, for instance, contain plenty of vitamin C, which is why a hot lemon and honey drink is traditionally used for treating colds.

Many plant foods also contain substances which have mild medicinal properties. These are good to include in a child's diet if he suffers from a particular health problem; specific foods are highlighted in the A to Z section of this book.

Babies weaned on plenty of fruit and vegetables often, as they grow older, continue to show a preference for these foods. Children who refuse to eat greens may be coaxed into drinking small quantities of freshly squeezed fruit and vegetable juices. Indeed, juices are a good way of topping up your child's intake of certain vitamins and minerals.

Opting for Organic

Organically grown or reared foods are the best choice for babies and young children. There is increasing concern over the health risks posed by pesticides sprayed on crops, fruits and vegetables, as well as over the drugs, antibiotics and unwholesome food given to livestock.

Amounts of pesticide residues considered to be safe for adults may be large enough to have an adverse effect on tiny infants. Furthermore, as they are fat-soluble these chemicals get stored away in the body's fatty tissue and accumulate over the years. Research suggests that pesticide residues have an adverse effect on the body's immune system. They may either suppress it – making us more vulnerable to viral and bacterial infections as well as opportunistic organisms such as the fungus Candida albicans (responsible for thrush) – or alter it, possibly leading to allergies or sensitivities to certain foods.

At high levels, pesticide residues have been linked with psychological and emotional problems such as depression, irritability, mood swings and impaired learning ability. While the precise risks to health are yet to be fully clarified, it is best to be on the safe side and limit your child's exposure to these chemicals as much as is feasibly possible. Happily, a nutrient-laden diet provides one of the best forms of protection from the harmful effects of pesticides and other environmental pollutants.

Between 4 and 6 months of age, introduce your baby gradually to (preferably organically grown) fresh fruits, vegetables and cereals. After 9 months you can add a little fresh fish, free range eggs and poultry and small quantities of meat from animals reared organically to your baby's diet. As children become older it may be harder to sustain an organic-only diet, but it definitely is worth including as much organically grown produce as possible.

Breastmilk – The Best Food for Babies

Breastmilk produced by a healthy mother is superior to any formula milk. It not only provides every nutrient in perfect balance with a growing baby's needs, but also endows your baby with an amazingly high resistance to infections. A baby nursed through most of his first year is continually supplied with antibodies that provide resistance to illnesses to which his mother has built up immunity. Fatty molecules present only in breastmilk also appear capable of destroying certain viruses and harmful bacteria.

Breastfeeding your baby is particularly recommended if allergies run in the family. Allergies are rare among breastfed babies, but are found in one in fifteen bottle-fed babies.

Mother's milk is enriched if she has a wholesome diet. The higher the mother's intake of protein, unsaturated fats, minerals and vitamins, the more of these nutrients will be present in breastmilk. Breastmilk is special in that it contains special long-chain polyunsaturated fatty acids (LCPUFAs), essential for the healthy development of the brain and with a role to play in intelligence and learning ability. These LCPUFAs are not present in cow's milk or infant formulas made from cow's milk and/or vegetable oils. Quantities of these fatty acids in breastmilk can be boosted by eating plenty of fatty fish such as mackerel, salmon and herrings. A nursing mother's requirement for the B complex vitamins, iron, calcium, and vitamin C increases while breastfeeding. You will need at least 300 mg a day for vitamin C to meet your baby's minimum requirement.

Fears that breastmilk contains pesticide residues should not put any mother off feeding her baby. You can control the pesticide derivatives in your milk by limiting the animal fats you eat prior to and while nursing. Avoid fatty cuts of meat. Opt for low-fat dairy products and supplement your diet with vegetable oils, nuts, avocados. Aerobic exercise also sweats out residues, and vitamin C neutralizes their harmful effects. Avoid strenuous dieting, however, as this uses up fat reserves – which you need while breastfeeding!

Ideally, babies should be breastfed for at least six months to derive maximum benefits, but even babies breastfed for six weeks enjoy many of the immune-enhancing benefits.

Ensuring Plentiful Milk for Baby

Most mothers find their milk supply dwindles if they are tired or emotionally upset. If you feel you do not have enough milk to satisfy your baby, nurse more often. Resist introducing a formula or solids, as this will only undermine your milk production even more. The more rest you get, the more milk you will have.

* Eat plenty of wholegrain cereals, fruits and vegetables, lean protein, and lots of fluids, especially apple and grape juice.
* Infusions of herbs such as Goat's rue, milkwort and borage are said to increase milk production. Pour 1 cup (240 ml) of boiling water over 1 teaspoon of dried leaves, infuse for 10 minutes and drink twice daily. Adding dill to your cooking can also help.
* Stress suppresses your milk supply – try meditation, massage and aromatherapy to relieve tension.
* The Homoeopathic remedy Agnus Castus 6c can be taken 4 times daily for up to 3 days.

Natural Sources of Vitamins and Minerals

Vitamin A	Milk, eggs, butter, cod liver oil. Best obtained from beta carotene. Carrots, spinach, cabbage, oranges and yellow fruits
Vitamin B_1 (Thiamin)	Wholegrains, pork, beef, peas, beans, lentils, brown rice
Vitamin B_2 (Riboflavin)	Milk, yoghurt, cereals, meat and some green leafy vegetables
Vitamin B_3 (Niacin)	Milk, fish, wholegrains, beef
Vitamin B_6 (Pyridoxine)	Meat, fish, egg yolk, wholegrain cereals, bananas, avocados, nuts, seeds and some green leafy vegetables
Vitamin B_5 (Pantothenic acid)	Eggs, wholegrain cereals and meat
Vitamin C	Most fruits and green vegetables, especially citrus fruits and blackcurrants as well as potatoes, green peppers and Brussels sprouts
Vitamin E	Vegetable oils, nuts, seeds, soya, lettuce, olives
Vitamin D	sunlight (on skin, stimulates synthesis of this nutrient); fatty fish, cod liver oil, eggs, milk, butter, cheese
Vitamin F (essential)	Vegetables, grains, beans, spinach, fatty acids, seafoods
Calcium	Milk, cheese, broccoli, legumes, green leafy vegetables, nuts, seeds, peas, beans, lentils, sesame seeds, chickpeas

Potassium	Fresh fruits and vegetables
Magnesium	Nuts, shrimp, soya beans, wholegrains and green leafy vegetables
Iron	Liver, egg yolk, cocoa, cane molasses, shellfish, parsley, poultry, nuts, green vegetables and wholemeal bread
Zinc	Meat (lamb, pork, beef), ginger root, split peas, lima beans, Brazil nuts, pecans, almonds, walnuts, egg yolk, wholewheat bread, rye, oats

Flower Remedies

Flower remedies are subtle elixirs for treating emotional and mental problems. They are invaluable for keeping babies and children happy and relaxed, providing one of the gentlest ways of relieving feelings of anxiety, fear, anger, irritability, etc. Flower remedies have a positive effect on babies and young children, who cannot be influenced by any so-called placebo effect – a fact that is often cited as proof of their potency.

Thousands of years ago, Australian Aborigines and Native Americans were using remedies made from flowers to ease emotional upsets. The healing power of flowers was then rediscovered and revived by Dr Edward Bach, a respected Harley Street physician specializing in pathology and bacteriology during the 1920s. Bach become disenchanted with a medicinal approach which focused on relieving the outward symptoms of an illness rather than searching for its true cause. He began his quest for a new healing system. Bach came to believe that the flowers blossoming in the fields and hedgerows of the British countryside could provide it.

Bach's 38 flower remedies are now renowned and widely used throughout the world. The first remedies he looked for were related to 12 key personality types. As personality traits reveal themselves at a very early age, you will be able to tell if your baby is, for instance, a Centuary type (kind, quiet, gentle, anxious to please) – or an Impatiens (always busy and rushing about, irritated by constraints, prone to tension and impatience). The most appropriate remedy for your child's personality is always worth having to hand to help him during times of change or upheaval.

The other 26 Bach Flower Remedies bring relief from different kinds of emotional discomfort and distress. You are likely to need different ones at different times.

More recently, other producers have introduced flower essences made from an extraordinarily diverse variety of flora – from modest hedgerow and alpine flowers to exotic orchids, antique roses and the blossoms of fruits such as avocado and bananas. Some flowers, especially those indigenous to the Australian Bush, Himalayan mountains and Hawaii, have a long tradition of being used in natural medicine. From this immense repertoire of flower essences are many that are particularly well-suited to treating the problems of babies and children.

How Flower Remedies Are Made

Dr Bach captured the flower's healing essence by floating freshly picked blooms in bowls of spring water and leaving them in sunlight on a cloudless day. This 'potentized' water was then mixed with brandy, which acted as a preservative. Most flower essences are still made in this way. Unlike aromatherapy oils and herbal medicines, these remedies do not contain any chemical substances. They are best described as a form of 'liquid energy'. They encapsulate the flower's healing energies and present it in a form that can be used therapeutically.

The Benefits of Flower Remedies

Infants are extremely impressionable. Rather like sponges, they soak up the atmosphere around them – making them far more susceptible to the disruptive influence of stress than most of us fully appreciate. Family tensions, parental arguments and so forth all affect them. Babies and young children also have their own stresses to deal with. Everything in a baby's life is new, and babies can become quite whingy and agitated when on the verge of major stages of development. Just like adults, they respond to stress by becoming tearful, angry, fretful or aggressive, although they cannot fathom out just why they feel this way – nor can they, of course, explain it to you. Walnut is very useful for babies and young children at such unsettling times and provides protection from disturbing outside influences. Star of Bethlehem helps to console children after a fright or sudden shock. It is recommended following a traumatic birth, accidents or any kind of unpleasant experience.

Floral Prescriptions

Well-chosen flower remedies may dispel temper tantrums and bring relief from nightmares. The link between psychological well-being and physical health is now well established. Children are much more likely to go down with a cold or other infection when they are feeling anxious, tense or worried. Many problems such as bedwetting and insomnia can also have a strong psychological component.

The beauty of flower remedies is that they are completely safe to use with no risk of any side-effects or adverse reactions. They are also easy to prescribe. Simply choose those essences whose qualities best match your child's emotional state at the time. With babies you will have to be fairly intuitive. Keep it simple: just one remedy at a time. As one problem clears, another may crop up a few months later, requiring a different flower remedy.

The remedies come in liquid form. Drops can be taken directly on the tongue, or can be added to a glass of spring water or fruit juice. They can also be added to the bath and are the ideal complement to essential oils.

Herbal Medicine

The medicinal use of herbs is probably as old as mankind itself. Almost every culture has its own version of herbal medicine, and in some countries these natural remedies are still used to treat many health problems. According to the World Health Organization, herbalism is three to four times more commonly practised throughout the world than conventional medicine.

Benefits of Herbal Remedies

Herbal remedies have a therapeutic action that is gentle and restorative. In addition to easing specific symptoms, they enhance the body's own natural healing capacity and so restore overall health and vitality.

The remedies are made from plants whose medicinal properties can be traced to the presence of various pharmacologically active ingredients. These constituents work in harmony to have the desired influence on the body. Many active ingredients have been 'copied' by drug companies to make orthodox medicines. A classic example is Willow Bark, a traditional remedy for headache and rheumatic pains. Its active principle is salicin, a chemical from which aspirin is derived. There are countless other examples, and scientific research continues into the chemical constituents of plants in order to isolate and synthesize substances with unique medicinal properties. Whereas antibiotics are ineffective against viruses, certain herbs such as Echinacea and Garlic appear to help the body resist and overcome viral infections.

Only the gentlest, most tried-and-tested herbal remedies are recommended for giving to babies and children at home. Because herbal remedies are made from the whole plant as found in nature, they are generally considered more gentle and less likely to cause adverse side-effects than chemically-synthesized medicines. And herbalists claim that the healing properties reside in the unique combination of chemical components present in the pure herb rather than in any one ingredient.

Many herbal remedies are often rich in particular vitamins and minerals. Rosehips, for instance, are an excellent source of vitamin C and bioflavonoids, while Dandelion root is rich in iron and potassium.

One of the safest ways to reap the benefits of herbs is to use them in cooking and salads. Familiar culinary herbs such as Thyme, Sage and Rosemary are strongly antiseptic.

Infusions of herbs make good natural medicines for babies and children. They can be sipped or given by the teaspoon, perhaps sweetened with a little honey to make them more enticing. An infusion of Chamomile or Lemon Balm before bedtime will help to ensure a good night's sleep. Raspberry leaves are excellent for soothing small children and infants; they can be used for diarrhoea, stomach upsets and for sore mouths.

Herbs are best when fresh. Some of the most useful herbs, such as Basil, Parsley and Thyme, can be grown in window boxes so they are always to hand. Freeze-dried organically grown herbs are another good option.

If something more sophisticated than a herb tea is required, tinctures and tablets are available from healthfood stores. For persistent or recurring health problems it is essential to consult a qualified herbal practitioner.

Herbal Preparations

INFUSIONS

A tisane or infusion is like a tea made from flowers, leaves and green stems. Use 1 tablespoon of dried herbs per pint (600 ml) of water, or 1 heaped teaspoon per cup. When using fresh herbs, double the quantity of herb can be used. Place the herbs in a pot or cup, pour on boiling water, cover and leave to stand (about four minutes for a tisane, up to 10 minutes for a stronger infusion). Strain. Herbal preparations can be taken hot or cold, and sweetened with honey to taste. Hot infusions tend to encourage perspiration and are helpful for treating colds, flu, fever and so forth.

DECOCTIONS

For berries, seeds, woody roots and barks of plants you will need to make a decoction. Place the herb or herbs in a saucepan, pour on some water, bring to the boil and then simmer for 10 to 15 minutes before straining. Use a glass, ceramic or enamel pan, not an aluminium one.

Use the same quantities as recommended for infusions, although you may need to add a little more water to allow for evaporation.

TINCTURES

Alcohol-based preparations are called tinctures. Ground or chopped herbs are left to steep in alcohol. Tinctures tend to be stronger volume for volume than infusions or decoctions. Dosages should be from 5 to 10 drops of tincture taken in a wineglass of just boiled water so the alcohol evaporates off in the steam. This should be left to stand until tepid, then given by the teaspoon or added to fruit juice or milk.

DOSAGES FOR INFUSIONS AND DECOCTIONS	
Newborn to 2 years	1 teaspoon
2 to 6 years	2 to 3 teaspoons
6 to 10 years	1 tablespoon

COMPRESSES AND POULTICES

To make a compress, use a clean cloth and soak it in a hot infusion or decoction. Place this while it is still as warm as possible upon the affected area. Change the compress when it cools down. The heat will enhance the activity of the herb.

To make a poultice, use either fresh or dried herbs. Apply the bruised leaves or root material of the fresh plant to the skin, either directly or between thin layers of gauze. When using dried herbs first make a paste by adding hot water, then apply in the same way as a compress. This is a good way to employ soothing herbs such as Comfrey Root or Slippery Elm.

CREAMS OR OINTMENTS

These contain a percentage of herbal infusion or tincture and are useful for helping wounds to heal and relieving skin conditions.

HERBAL RECIPES

These are recommended for various ailments listed in the A – Z section of this book, and are listed here for your quick reference.

Cream for Drawing Out Glass, Thorns and Splinters
* 30 ml Rescue Remedy Cream
* $1/2$ teaspoon Slippery Elm powder
* $1/2$ teaspoon Marshmallow Root tincture
* 1 teaspoon Calendula lotion or oil

Mix ingredients together and apply to affected area. Wait at least 2 hours before attempting to extract the thorn, splinter or bit of glass.

Elderflower Syrup for Coughs, Colds and Flu
* Fresh elderflowers
* Vegetable glycerine
* Elderberries (where available)

Fill a jam jar with freshly picked elderflowers, cover with vegetable glycerine and leave to stand in the sun for a day. Strain. When berries are in season (in the Autumn), you can add these to the jar when the petals have settled; leave in the sun again, ideally for a few days before straining and bottling. Keep refrigerated until needed (it will keep for up to two years).

Little Ones' Cough Syrup
* Vegetable glycerine
Tinctures of:
* Marshmallow Root
* Lobelia
* Balm of Gidead buds
* Elderflowers
* Elderberries

To approximately 30 ml of vegetable glycerine, add $1/2$ teaspoon of Lobelia and 1 teaspoon of each of the others tinctures, stirring well all the time to ensure they are evenly distributed throughout the mixture.

Children's Stress Formula

Tinctures of:
* Borage
* Chamomile
* Lemon Balm
* Liquorice
* St John's Wort
* Skullcap
* Wild Oat

Children's Immunity Formula

Tinctures of:
* Astragalus
* Echinacea
* Liquorice
* Marshmallow Root
* Raspberry leaves
* Red Clover
* Rosehips
* St John's Wort

Immune Balance Formula

Tinctures of:
* Astragalus
* Marshmallow Root
* Raspberry
* St John's Wort

Happy Child Formula

Tinctures of:
* Catmint
* Chamomile
* Dandelion Root
* Lavender
* Liquorice
* Lobelia
* Peppermint
* Red Clover
* Rosehips
* Skullcap
* Vervain

Method of Preparation

For each remedy, add 1 teaspoon of each of the tinctures listed to a small glass dropper bottle and shake well. Add 5 drops (for babies up to 12 months old) or 10 drops (for children over 1 year old) to 6 fl oz/180 ml of mineral water, fruit juice or milk.

Some ready-prepared formulas are available from the Sunflower Vital Health Initiative and Herbs Hands Healing (*see Further Addresses*).

SAFETY TIPS

Although herbalism is a natural form of healing, it is not entirely harmless. Herbs have a strong therapeutic value and, like conventional medications, can have side-effects. For this reason herbs must be used with respect and common sense.

Always be cautious, especially when treating babies and children. If any problem does not respond to simple herbal remedies after two or three days you should take your child to a qualified practitioner.

It is unwise to continue using herbs over a prolonged period of time, or to exceed the recommended safe dosage.

Homoeopathy

Homoeopathy is a system of medicine that treats a whole pattern of symptoms. It considers all the emotional and mental changes associated with an illness, as well as the physical ones. Thus the most effective remedy is the one which matches a person's 'symptom picture' as closely as possible.

Principles of Homoeopathy

Based on the ancient Greek doctrine that 'like cures like', today's remedies were largely discovered by a German physician called Samuel Hahnemann in the early 19th century. He regarded the medicine of his day, which featured blood-letting and purging, to be harsh and crude. He searched for gentler and safer means of treating illness.

Hahnemann's idea was inspired by the discovery that a herbal remedy for malaria, the cinchona tree bark, actually produced the symptoms of the disease, such as headache and fever, when taken by a healthy person. He concluded that symptoms were the body's way of fighting illness and that medicines producing the same symptoms as a given illness could also help recovery. It was later found that cinchona bark contains quinine, the first drug used against malaria.

Hahnemann felt that small doses of homoeopathic remedies would be safer than large ones, yet still remain effective. Many homoeopathic remedies are so diluted that they contain very few molecules of the original substance. All the remedies are made from naturally occurring substances, mostly of plant and mineral origin. Each remedy is carefully tested (according to a system known as 'proving') on volunteers, who take a very dilute remedy and record all their symptoms in detail for up to a year. This includes its effects on sleeping and eating habits, moods and relationships, as well as on any physical symptoms.

Homoeopathic remedies can be highly effective and offer viable alternatives to orthodox drugs. Many conventional doctors are also qualified homoeopaths, and there are now several homoeopathic hospitals in Britain run by the NHS.

Diagnosing for Babies and Children

Choosing the right remedy is not always straightforward. There are, for instance, over 100 possible remedies for treating hay fever. To select the most appropriate homoeopathic remedy you have to be extremely observant and note every kind of symptom as well as changes in your child's behaviour, no matter how minor these may seem.

Three children suffering from hay fever may all have the classic symptoms – sneezing, runny nose and swollen eyes – yet each will require a different remedy. The first may have a burning throat and feel restless, worried and exhausted: in this case you would give Arsenicum album; the second may have itching in the ears and a headache, and be irritable: Nux vomica; the third may have a cough which makes the eyes water and may feel depressed and touchy: Natrum muriaticum.

Parents often feel their child has undergone a personality change when he is ill or coming down with something. These mental changes are extremely important to take into account. Some homoeopathic prescriptions are based almost entirely on these changes.

Alterations in appetite, food preferences and so forth are all symptoms called modalities in homoeopathy and are of great importance when trying to choose the correct remedy.

The remedies recommended in this book are those that tend to come up time and time again in reference to a particular ailment. It is beyond the scope of this book to describe each one in detail, so if you would like more specific information about a particular remedy you might want to refer to the References and Further Reading chapter (*page 288*), which lists other books on the subject.

Giving Homoeopathic Remedies

Remedies are best given individually so you can gauge each one's effects. The remedies were all originally proved separately, so it is not known how they interact if mixed. The more the remedy is diluted and succussed (shaken), the stronger it becomes as a cure. The more precise the match-up is with your child's symptoms, the higher the potency can be. For those with little experience in homoeopathy the 6c, 12c and 30c potencies are the best ones to use. You should only use 30c when you are quite sure you have got the remedy that precisely covers the major symptoms, including those concerning your child's disposition.

For intense and acute symptoms, several doses will be needed. In the case of fever or pain you may need to give one dose every hour for several doses until there is lasting relief. If relief comes after one to three doses, stop giving the remedy – your child will probably continue to get better. If relief is noticeable, but slight, give two or three more doses. 'Relief' in these cases could take the form of your child simply being less ratty or sleeping better. If there is no relief at all after three or four doses, the remedy you have chosen is not the right one.

Homoeopathic tablets come in various forms:

* Soft tablets dissolve quickly and easily under the tongue and are easily crushed for administering to babies.

* Hard tablets can be crushed between two spoons and sprinkled onto the tongue (thus making it difficult for your child to spit the remedy out). You can also dissolve the crushed tablet in a little mineral water, stir vigorously and give a teaspoon at a time.

* Liquid potencies can be made up for children known to be allergic to cow's milk. The remedy is supplied in dropper bottles and can be dropped onto the tongue for babies and children.

* Creams and ointments contain homoeopathic amounts

of the substance in a base for use on cuts, rashes, stings and so forth.

When giving your child a tablet, carefully tip it into the lid of the bottle, transfer it to the palm of your child's hand or directly onto the tongue, then replace the lid. Try never to touch the tablets unnecessarily.

Never put back tablets that have fallen on the floor or anywhere else, as they will contaminate the others. It is best not to eat, drink (except water) or brush teeth for 10 to 20 minutes before and after taking a remedy, although remedies given to toddlers who have eaten before and after still seem to work.

Homoeopathic remedies will keep their strength for years without deteriorating. They should be stored in a cool dark place with their tops screwed on tightly, away from strong-smelling substances such as peppermint, eucalyptus or coffee. Don't keep them in the bathroom cabinet next to perfumes or essential oils!

Useful Homoeopathic Creams and Ointments

* Calendula (marigold) – helps to heal wounds, especially effective for dry, cracked or scratched skin. Good for burns, scalds, cuts and scratches, eczema and skin rashes.
* Urtica urens (nettle) – helps to relieve the itching of eczema and any form of rash.
* Hypericum (St John's Wort) -- soothes and heals especially where nerves have been damaged. For burns

including sunburn, cuts, wounds and insect bites.
* Hypercal – a mixture of Calendula and Hypericum for soothing and healing wounds. For cuts, inflammations and injuries.

Consulting a Professional Homoeopath

Some chronic conditions such as allergies, asthma and eczema may need treatment with what is known as a *constitutional* remedy, which is best prescribed by a professional homoeopath.

A constitutional remedy aims to strengthen the immune system and decrease susceptibility to illness. A child's constitution is his genetic inheritance tempered or modified by environment. A strong constitution can withstand considerable pressure without feeling ill, while a weak constitution (or immune system) has far greater susceptibility to illness. In an epidemic not everyone will be affected, but only those who are most susceptible.

The correctly chosen constitutional remedy works by strengthening the body's vitality and its ability to respond to stress. Homoeopaths believe there is a balancing mechanism – Hahnemann called it 'the vital force' – which keeps us in health provided the stresses on our constitution are not too great nor long-lived. Symptoms are simply the body's way of telling us how it is coping with stress, so they should not be suppressed. Constitutional remedies are given to stimulate the vital force and clear any lasting effects of past illnesses, vaccinations and so forth.

Hydrotherapy

The healing power of water has been valued since ancient times for enhancing health as well as relieving specific ailments. The ancient Chinese and Native Americans knew of the therapeutic effect of water, as did the ancient Greeks and Romans. Many Greek temples were built on the sites of hot water springs renowned for their beneficial healing properties.

Today water therapy is still highly valued for its health-giving properties and plays a pivotal role at spas throughout Europe, especially in France and Italy.

Hydrotherapy is also an important part of Naturopathy (*see page 47*).

The Benefits of Hydrotherapy

Water can be used in a variety of ways to induce relaxation, stimulate circulation, promote cleansing and rekindle vitality. Temperature has an important bearing on the effect of water.

BATHS

Spending 10 to 20 minutes in a warm bath is wonderfully therapeutic, relieving tension, easing pain and encouraging the elimination of impurities from the body. A therapeutic soak is also an excellent way of treating skin complaints.

Salt Water

The healing power of sea water is legendary. It is good for most skin conditions as it helps to promote cleansing and encourage healing.

Epsom salts drive off chills and colds.

Oatmeal or Bran

Raw oatmeal or bran (tied up in muslin or thin cotton) is thought to be helpful in clearing up eczema and other skin complaints. Adding essential oils to the bath brings additional benefits.

SPRAY TREATMENTS

These are not generally recommended for children as they have a powerful effect on the body. Gentle showering of certain areas, however, is safe and will gently boost the circulation.

INHALATIONS

Hot steamy vapours are cleansing and relaxing. They can be used to treat respiratory problems, blocked nasal passages and catarrh on the chest, especially when a few drops of eucalyptus, pine or thyme essential oil are added to the water.

Croup in children and bouts of coughing are also eased by breathing in steamy air.

COLD WRAPS

Good for reducing inflammation and burning sensations. They can be used for skin disorders, colds and feverishness. A sheet wrung out in cold water is wrapped around the body. A dry sheet and a warm blanket are in turn wrapped over the wet sheet. A hot water bottle may be needed to keep the feet warm. The wrap is removed when the wet sheet dries out and the body is then sponged with tepid water and rubbed dry with a fresh towel.

Water from Within

The importance of drinking plenty of pure water cannot be overemphasized. Water is nature's cleanser and revitalizer. Our bodies are 70 per cent water, as is the planet we live on. We need water to help cells to replace themselves, enable food to be digested properly and cleanse all our tissues. There are times when children need to drink extra quantities of water to maintain healthy body fluids. Children lose water through their skin, more so during hot weather and after exercise. Water needs to be constantly replenished to avoid any possibility of dehydration.

Ideally children should drink up to 1 litre of pure spring water a day – more during the hot weather.

Squashes and fizzy drinks should be discouraged as they do not have the same thirst-quenching or cleansing benefits. Indeed, as they are invariably laden with sugar or artificial sweeteners, drunk on a regular basis they increase the risk of tooth decay, upset the body's electrolyte balance and fill your child's body with empty calories.

AQUA VITAE

For guaranteed purity always opt for mineral waters, but check the salt content – *Evian* is one of the few that is considered suitable for babies.

Mineral waters with high salt/mineral content have more of a diuretic effect and can place stress on the kidneys.

If drinking tap water, always filter it first to remove traces of pesticides, nitrates and other impurities, then boil to evaporate off the chlorine.

Do not regularly give water with more than 1.5 mg of fluoride per litre to babies or children, as it can cause mottling or weakening of the teeth.

Massage

Massage is one of the oldest forms of healing. It was practised in the Middle and Far East over 5,000 years ago. Physicians in ancient Greece were also skilled in the art of massage. In the 5th century BC, Hippocrates ('the Father of Medicine'), wrote that 'the way to health is to have a scented bath and an oiled massage each day.'

The Benefits of Massage

Massage, even in its simplest forms, has an enormously beneficial influence on both emotional and physical well-being.

Nothing is as comforting and reassuring as the sympathetic touch of a hand.

In the early years touch seems to play a vital role in the healthy development of babies and young children. Those who look after premature babies have noted that the ones who are gently stroked are more likely to thrive than those deprived of touch. In one hospital study, babies in incubators developed their lung capacity much more quickly if they were touched or stroked by their parents than did those who were handled only by the nurses or left alone.

A child who is cuddled and stroked grows up feeling loved and secure. Massage works in much the same way, and is a marvellous tool for enhancing empathy and strengthening the bond between parent and child, and building up the child's feelings of confidence and self-esteem. Young children need masses of attention; a massage can be an opportunity for you to devote your full attention and affection to your child, something both of you can look forward when made into part of a daily or weekly routine.

As well as relieving tensions, massage helps to restore a sense of calm and balance, especially after any shock or trauma. Children are particularly susceptible to stress, perhaps more so than adults because everything is new and life is constantly changing.

A regular body massage also enhances physical health and vitality. Stroking relaxes and tones the muscles, promotes healthy blood circulation and stimulates lymphatic drainage to ensure swift removal of wastes from the body. It is good for the skin, especially when vegetable oils such as sweet almond, grapeseed, avocado and sunflower are used (individually or as a base oil for essential oils).

Gently massaging specific areas can ease colic, relieve headaches and treat insomnia. Massage will also speed recovery after an illness and is a valuable aid to convalescence.

Massage for Babies

Newborn babies respond well to touch, but they probably won't enjoy a proper massage. Massaging a new baby begins with caressing and fondling. After getting to know your baby in the early days you may then wish to use a few simple massage movements.

Sit on the floor with your legs stretched out in front of you. Place a soft towel on your lap. Place baby down on his front, his head facing your tummy and turned to one side. Put a few drops of massage oil in the palms of your hands and rub them together. Place your hands on baby's buttocks, fingers pointing away from you. With very light pressure, draw your hands towards you, bringing them gently up baby's back to the shoulder. Using your middle and ring fingers only, return down the sides of baby's body to the buttocks. Repeat several times.

Lift baby up and draw your knees up towards you. Nestle baby on your thighs, supporting his head with your knees. Hold one of baby's hands to stop him wriggling around; lightly rest the fingers of your other hand on baby's tummy. Using the flat surface of your fingers, draw clockwise circles around his tummy, being as gentle as possible.

BABY'S MASSAGE OIL FORMULA	
Chamomile	1 drop
Lavender	1 drop
Geranium	1 drop
	Diluted in 30 ml of sweet almond oil

Although single essences are generally recommended for babies, this formula is particularly useful as it helps to treat eczema and cradle cap, soothes during times of teething problems and strengthens the immune defences.

Massaging Toddlers and Older Children

As your child gets older and more fidgety you need to adapt your technique slightly. It may only be possible to do parts of the body, such as the hands, feet and tummy, at any one time. A full body massage may have to be reserved for a weekend treat.

* Back massage – good for relaxation, insomnia, aches and pains, shoulder tension and breathing difficulties
* Foot and hand massage – helps poor circulation, cold feet and skin conditions; acts as a general tonic (*see Reflexology, page 51*).
* Tummy massage – for anxiety and all kinds of digestive upsets including colic, nausea and wind
* Scalp massage – for eczema, cradle cap, headaches, insomnia and to promote general relaxation.

How to Massage

The best time and place for massage is before or after a morning or evening bath for babies. Toddlers and young children may be most receptive to massage when winding down for sleep. Make sure the time you choose is also good for you. A child will sense if you are tense, rushed, angry or irritable, and will feel uncomfortable about being massaged. He may even come to think of massage as a chore you feel obliged to perform – this can only be counter-productive.

A duvet on the floor becomes a mini-bed with pillows or cushions, a good base for massage. Place a pillow under your child's head and cover his body with a towel or a soft blanket. Remove any jewellery you have on and make sure that your nails are short and clean and that your hands are warm.

Maintain contact with your child's body at all times. Use very light pressure – featherweight for newborns, becoming more and more firm as your child matures. There are no hard-and-fast rules; it is best for massage to be rhythmic and free-flowing.

Massage Strokes

* Stroking (also known as *Effleurage*)

    Slow, stroking movements form the basis of a massage and are the ones you will use most. They are usually performed with the hands close together, thumbs about 2.5 cm/1 inch apart. Long, sweeping movements are warming and relaxing. Brisk movements are invigorating and stimulating.

* Kneading (*Petrissage*)

    Use your fingers and thumbs to squeeze and roll the flesh very gently as if kneading dough. Use only on shoulders or very fleshy areas, and sparingly, to stretch and relax tense muscles.

* Friction

    Small circling movements with the fingers, pads of the thumbs or heel of the hands, to help relax muscles.

* Pressuring

    Using the pads of your thumbs or forefingers, apply pressure to certain areas such as around the shoulders or at either side of the spine. You could work on relevant acupressure points during this massage.

When Not to Massage

* Never massage a child who has a fever or is infectious, as he will be hot and aching.
* Avoid massaging cut or bruised areas.
* Never massage new scar tissue – wait until the skin is no longer red and sore.
* If your child has had a recent fracture or break, wait at least two months before massaging the area.

Naturopathy

Since the earliest days, when it was known as the 'nature cure', naturopathy has intended to stimulate and support the body's own self-healing powers.

Although the term was first used only at the beginning of the 20th century, the principles date back at least to 400 BC when Hippocrates became famous for his treatment of disease in accordance with natural laws. He felt that cures should work *with* the body and be as natural as possible. Naturopathy employs foods – especially fruits and vegetables – water and various other natural elements to encourage the body to heal itself.

Principles of Naturopathy

Naturopathy sees illness as a disturbance in the body's normal balance. When, for whatever reason, health breaks down naturopathy sets out to identify the underlying cause. The particular type of illness may be the result of various bacteria, viruses, allergies or external factors, but a naturopath will be more concerned with why the person has succumbed to them. In other words, a naturopath will want to know what is responsible for someone's weakness and lack of resistance.

Diagnosis is directed towards finding out why health has broken down in the first place. This is rather like piecing together a jigsaw. A naturopath aims to identify each person's strengths, weaknesses and individual needs, and to assess the quality of his or her lifestyle and environment.

Naturopathic Therapies

Naturopathy holds that the body has the power to heal itself, given the right environment. The therapies aim to create this healthy environment. They include a wholesome diet, hydrotherapy, massage, osteopathy, relaxation and possibly even herbal preparations. As symptoms are seen as a positive sign that the body is dealing with a particular illness or fighting an infection, naturopathy does not try to suppress them.

Sometimes symptoms are temporarily aggravated during treatment. This is what is known, in naturopathy, as a 'healing crisis'. It indicates that the healing process is underway.

Care is taken to ensure that symptoms do not overcome the person's reserves of energy or hinder the body's ability to make a good recovery.

THE NATUROPATHIC DIET

The basic diet is known as the reform diet. It suggests that everyone should eat at least five helpings of fresh fruit or vegetables each day. Refined carbohydrate such as cakes, biscuits and sweets are limited to two or three portions each week.

Fresh juices, preferably apple and grape, diluted with water should be drunk twice a day.

* Hydrotherapy – plays an important role in the naturopath's therapeutic repertoire.
* Naturopathic osteopathy – a professional naturopath may apply gentle neuromuscular stimulation to areas of the body where symptoms have appeared or to specific points related to them. At home you can use massage.
* Compresses – for bruises, bites, skin problems and so forth.
* To make a hot compress – useful for muscular aches and pains, bruises, psoriasis, eczema, etc.: Fill a small bowl with hot water (you can add 1–2 drops of a relevant essential oil). Make a pad from clean white cotton material and place on the surface of the water.

Squeeze lightly and apply to the affected area. Keep in place with ordinary cling film.

* To make a cold compress – useful for insect bites, sprains, inflammation, headaches and swelling: As above, but use cold water with ice cubes added.

Osteopathy

Osteopathy is a treatment given by fully trained professionals and is not something you can do at home. As many childhood health problems – ranging from asthma and colic to sleeplessness and hyperactivity – can be relieved by this treatment, it may be recommended in certain instances to work in conjunction with other self-help natural remedies.

Osteopathy is concerned with the balance and alignment of the whole body structure – the bones, joints, muscles, ligaments and other supportive soft tissue.

It was founded by an American doctor, Andrew Taylor Still, in the mid-1870s. His detailed knowledge of human anatomy, combined with his earlier study of engineering, made him interested in the body as a machine. He became certain that many illnesses arise when part of the body's structure gets out of alignment, as a result of injury or stress, for example. He discovered that manipulation could be used to correct physical imbalances and so alleviate illness.

Stuart Korth, co-founder of the Osteopathic Centre for Children in London, feels that all newborn babies would benefit from being checked over by an osteopath after birth, even if it was a 'normal' delivery (i.e., without complications). This is even more important if the baby has been born with the umbilical cord wrapped around his neck or delivered by forceps. Unresolved mechanical strain experienced at birth has been found to lead to nervous disorders in infancy and behavioural problems in childhood.

As babies become ever more mobile and adventurous, the odd tumble is inevitable. However, bumps and jolts (as after falling downstairs or falling out of the cot) can lead to bodily imbalances, and these may set the scene for other health problems.

Emotional stress such as anxiety and apprehension can be translated into physical tensions which may also have a role to play in creating imbalance.

A professional osteopath will want to know about any such physical traumas and emotional distress when trying to trace the underlying cause of a health problem.

Case History

Kerry was $2^1/_2$ years old when she had her first asthma attack. Her GP prescribed an inhaler, but before using it her mother decided to take Kerry to the Osteopathic Centre for Children. During consultation her osteopath discovered that Kerry had been kicked very hard in the back by a young boy at nursery a year earlier. Afterwards Kerry had developed a kidney infection which had been treated with antibiotics. Her osteopath could still feel a great deal of residual tension in the area of Kerry's chest and diaphragm. She also discovered a history of asthma in the family, so there was a genetic predisposition waiting to be unleashed.

After five treatments to release the tension and restore balance, Kerry stopped having asthma attacks and showed no need for an inhaler. Her mother remains vigilant and, should the symptoms reappear, she is determined to take Kerry for follow-up osteopathic treatment.

Cranial Osteopathy

Cranial manipulation is part and parcel of a thorough osteopathic treatment. The cranium is the dome of bone protecting the brain. It is not made up of one continuous piece but of eight separate bones which have hairline cracks between them. Once it was felt that these bones were immovable after childhood, but it is now known that they can move very slightly in relation to one another. They move most at birth, and if they do not return to their proper position afterwards they can distort the flow of 'shock absorber' fluid around the brain, resulting in pressure on parts of the body via nerves originating in the brain. Later in life, blows to the head can cause similar problems.

Cranial osteopathy aims to detect and correct pressures and displacements in the skull and facial bones, using a delicate form of manipulation. The touch may be barely perceptible, consisting of tapping, 'moulding' and holding the bones to coax them into the proper alignment.

Reflexology

Reflexology is a sort of pressure massage applied to the hands and feet. It was certainly being practised over 2,000 years ago by the Ancient Egyptians and Chinese, and is still used today by millions of people throughout world. Reflexology is based on the idea that every area of the body is mapped out on the soles of our feet and palms of our hands. Our hands and feet can be likened to windows that enable us to reach into the body. Massaging them is a simple and straightforward way of achieving better health.

The Benefits of Reflexology

Precisely how reflexology works has not yet been established, but pressure sensors on the feet are thought to relay messages to associated areas of the body. Reflexology is thought to be helpful in treating a number of different ailments. Research studies have found it to have a positive effect on several common childhood conditions such as bedwetting, diarrhoea, bronchitis and infantile asthma. It may even help to treat ear infections.

Using a special kind of thumb pressure, reflexologists slowly work over the surface of the feet and/or hands. Reflex points that are tender or sore when touched indicate a tension or congestion in the corresponding region of the body. Knowing which systems are not working efficiently gives greater insight into the underlying cause of health problems. Massaging and kneading these sensitive spots also helps to tone up the relevant sluggish systems.

Anyone can practise reflexology. You simply need to familiarize yourself with the zones on the feet and hands that correspond to particular areas of the body.

While a professional may use reflexology as a means of diagnosis, for those without much experience it is best used as a relaxing and rebalancing treatment.

Babies seem to like reflexology. A gentle foot or hand massage is also one of the most effective ways of settling a restless baby.

Children are often fascinated by the idea of massaging a certain part of the foot to soothe a tummy ache or relieve an attack of hay fever. They can also learn to do reflexology for themselves, a valuable self-help tool that they can use throughout life.

To work properly, reflexology needs to be done on a regular basis. At first a young child may wriggle away when you take hold of his feet. Try to acclimatize him slowly. Casually picking up a child's foot and working with it while focusing his attention on something else, for instance while watching a video, or making reflexology into a game is a good way to start. The younger they are when you start (preferably before the age of 2), the better.

How to Give a Reflexology Treatment

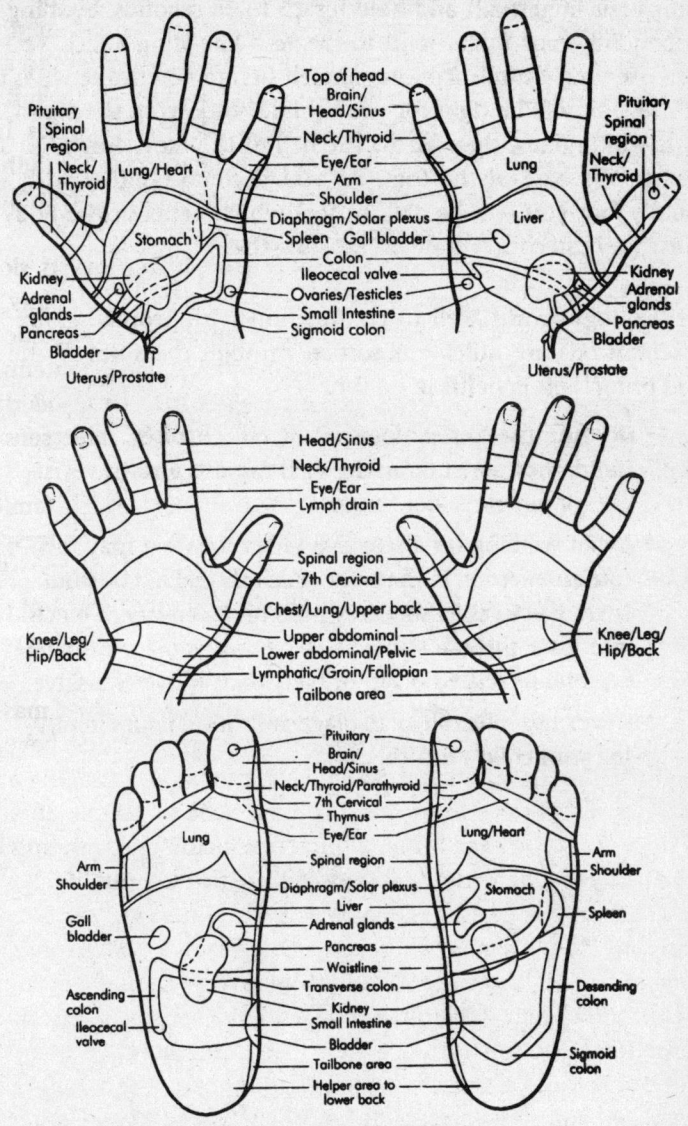

FIGURE 2: REFLEXOLOGY ZONES OF THE HANDS AND FEET

Apply firm pressure with your fingertips (but without digging in with your fingernail) and hold for 15 to 30 seconds, bending and unbending your finger joint to create a kneading effect. You can also use your thumb. Try on yourself first to determine what kind of pressure will be right for your child. Work from the big toe out to the little ones, then across the ball of the foot, down the sides and to the base of the foot. As you become familiar with your child's foot you will be able to feel which areas in the body are tense and can concentrate on relaxing them.

Reflexology works well in conjunction with aromatherapy. The essential oils are quickly absorbed through the soles of the feet and bring their benefits in no time.

* Do not use reflexology on a cut, bruises, injured hand, foot, wrist or ankle, or if there is a rash, verrucae, or athlete's foot fungus.
* Avoid working on a sensitive reflex area – it may indicate an infection in the body which should not be stimulated. If your child suddenly pulls his foot away or bursts into tears, this can signify that the area you are working on (and its related organ or body part) is over-sensitive.
* Never use reflexology to diagnose critical issues involving your child's health.

Relaxation, Rest and Sleep

Sleep is one of nature's best healers. The instinct to sleep when we feel unwell is in-built and can work wonders for reviving babies and children. Those who appear to be sickening for something often seem to shake off an illness after a good long sleep, waking up bright and cheerful again.

When the body is at rest all its energies can be channelled into fighting off an infection or restoring a healthy equilibrium. Today illness is often regarded as an inconvenience and children are not always encouraged to have the rest they need to fight off infections and make a full recovery. The body's self-healing mechanism takes time to work – the immune system can take up to eight weeks to regain strength after a simple cold virus. As well as getting enough sleep, babies and children with a tummy ache or cold need time to rest and take it easy.

In the long run, a well-rested child will regain vibrant health and emerge with better resistance to other ills (such as coughs and colds) than one who is dosed up with paracetamol or antibiotics and sent back to school too soon.

Minor bugs, tummy aches and fevers often come at the moment when babies and toddlers are making developmental leaps, for instance just as they are on the verge of sitting up, crawling, walking or talking for the first time. At these times they need peace and quiet so they can adjust to the changes that are taking place.

Sufficient sleep is also important to maintaining good health. An over-tired child becomes grumpy and grizzley, which can in itself lead to ill-health. Plenty of sleep at night and perhaps an hour's nap in the day can make all the difference to temperament and behaviour, especially for pre-school children.

Rest is also essential for a child's growth and development. If children are weary and fractious it is far better to let them drop off to sleep, even if it is not an ideal time. They can always eat or go out to play later.

Of course some children have a remarkable ability to stay awake even if they are incredibly tired. Any kind of exercise, such as a long walk in the fresh air can work wonders for bringing on sleep. A bath with soothing essential oils can also be conducive to sleep.

The Art of Relaxation

Like adults, children may suffer from stress and need time to themselves so they can relax and unwind. We now know that stress has a highly deleterious influence on health. It undermines the body's immune defences and increases susceptibility to all kinds of illness. Care should be taken not to create too much upheaval in children's lives and to shield them from adult topics of conversation which can be a source of anxiety for them. They should certainly be spared the sort of stress an adult has to handle.

Relaxation Techniques for Children

Switching off is a wonderful way of relieving tensions in the mind and body. Children who learn the art of relaxation at an early age will be equipped with an invaluable tool for preserving their sense of well-being throughout life.

* listening to music – try tapes with songs specially designed for children
* reading and listening to stories
* visualization – children have wonderful imaginations and are very good at daydreaming, which is the mind's natural way of finding tranquillity when life gets stressful. You can help them to enter their own dreamland with guided visualization. To begin they must shut their eyes, then you should guide them to a magical place where they can find stillness and security.

It can be somewhere already visited or an imaginary place. The only rule is always to conjure up cozy images and happy events.

* meditation – this relaxation technique is for slightly older children who have learned to focus their attention. Meditation sounds complicated but it is incredibly simple. It is best if you do it with your child until he acquires this skill. Both of you should sit still, shut your eyes and simply focus on breathing slowly in and out for 10 to 15 minutes.

The Natural Medicine Chest

Various remedies are always useful and are good to have handy:

Aromatherapy	Essential oils of Chamomile, Lavender, Tea Tree and Eucalyptus
Diet and nutritional therapy	Vitamin C with bioflavanoids (250 mg tablets) Multi-vitamin and mineral supplements. Bifidophilus powder (acidophilus and bifidus bacteria)
Flower Remedies	Rescue Remedy (Bach Flower Remedies) Five Flower (Healing Herbs) Remedy. Other options are First Aid Essence (Findhorn Flower Essences or Jan de Vries' Emergency Essence)
Herbal Remedies	Echinacea tincture Garlic capsules

                    Aloe Vera juice or gel
                    Crystallized ginger
                    Slippery Elm powder

Homoeopathy Arnica tablets and cream
                    Aconite tablets
                    Chamomilla drops
                    Calendula cream and/or tablets
                    Hypericum cream

Part Two

A – Z of Childhood Ailments

A TO Z OF CHILDHOOD AILMENTS

*Please note that throughout this A–Z
the most pertinent remedies for each ailment
are marked with an asterisk (*).*

A

ABDOMINAL PAIN *See* STOMACH ACHE

ACCIDENTS AND INJURIES

Prevention is the best cure for accidents. All parents learn to be vigilant, usually foreseeing potentially hazardous situations and steering children away from them. No matter how observant you are, however, accidents do happen from time to time. Fortunately most accidents are minor and can be dealt with by using the recommended remedies.

Homoeopathy

* Arnica is the number one remedy for accidents, injuries, trauma and shock. Taken early it will reduce

shock, swelling and bruising. Give 1 dose of the 30C potency immediately, and 1 a day for the next 2 days.

* Arnica ointment – apply as soon as possible to the affected area (on unbroken skin only). You can also use Arnica lotion applied on a piece of lint or gauze and kept in place until the swelling has subsided.

* Hypercal cream or ointment – a blend of Calendula and Hypericum, this helps to soothe and heal cuts, wounds and injuries.

Aromatherapy

* Lavender is one of the best essential oils for treating wounds of all kinds.

* For babies over 6 months old: Lavender or Eucalyptus

* For children over 1 year old: Lavender, Eucalyptus, Tea Tree or Geranium. Add the appropriate number of drops (*see page 6*) to a base of Almond or Rosehip oil.

To ease pain, reduce swelling and encourage healing, gently massage your chosen aromatherapy oil into the wound or affected area morning and evening.

Other Helpful Remedies

Naturopathy

* Wrap some crushed ice in a flannel and apply to the injured area.

Flower Remedies

* Rescue Remedy (Bach Flower Remedies), Five Flower Remedy (Healing Herbs) or First Aid Flower Essence (Findhorn Flower Essences). Give 2 drops on the

tongue every hour until your child is calm, and 2 drops a day until the injury has healed.

* Jacaranda (Australian Bush Essences) – a helpful preventative for children who are accident prone, always rushing about, aimless and/or 'scatty'.

Professional Therapy

Osteopathy

Unless there is an obvious injury like a fracture, physical traumas often have no repercussions once the pain and swelling have subsided. However, sometimes bumps and jolts can throw the body out of alignment, albeit subtly. They may even lie at the root of health problems which appear several months or even years later for no apparent reason. The earlier imbalances are corrected, the better. After any severe bump such as falling down stairs, it is worth seeing an osteopath for an examination, if only for peace of mind.

Doctor's Prescription

Medical intervention is necessary for large or deep wounds, any sign of infection (swelling, inflammation and pus), and when there is an injury to the head.

See also **Bruises, Cuts and Scratches**

ACHES AND PAINS

The term 'growing pains' is often used to cover the aches and pains children experience for no apparent reason. Sometimes they come at night and go by the morning, especially aches in the arms and legs. Aches may simply be the result of too much exercise or overtaxing the body physically.

Aromatherapy/Massage

* Lavender and Peppermint are helpful for easing aches and pains.

* For children over 6 years old: Lavender, Peppermint or Rosemary, or a simple blend of any two of these essences. Gently rub and massage the affected area.

Hydrotherapy

Fill the bath with warm water deep enough to cover your child's shoulders. Add 1 teaspoon of the recommended aromatherapy oil, swirling the water round to make sure it is evenly dispersed.

Your child should remain in this bath for at least 15 minutes.

Professional Therapies

Osteopathy

Aches and pains are often a sign of residual tension in certain areas of the body which can be relieved by professional osteopathic treatment.

Homoeopathy

A professional homoeopath can prescribe specific remedies for growing pains.

Herbal Remedies

A herbalist may recommend an infusion of Meadowsweet, or Boneset tincture. Either of these can be used safely at home.

Doctor's Prescription

If a child complains of a pain continuing in the same place for a long time, you should take him to the doctor. Joint pain needs special attention as it may be due to an infection or inflammation.

ALLERGIES

An allergy may be described as an inappropriate response to a particular substance or chemical involving the immune system.

Allergies tends to run in families, so if either mother or father suffers from asthma, eczema, hay fever, etc., your child may be predisposed to having allergic reactions.

Many everyday things can cause allergies, but what affects one person does not necessarily provoke a reaction in another.

Some of the most common allergens are grass pollen, dust, house dust mites, animal fur and fluff (dander), dairy products, wheat, perfumes, and food additives and preservatives.

An allergic reaction occurs when these foreign substances get into the bloodstream via the skin or mucous membranes lining the nose, lungs and intestinal tract, where they trigger an excessive biochemical response. The typical allergic symptoms are caused by a number of different chemicals, most particularly histamine.

Typical Symptoms

A congested or runny nose, itchy and watering eyes, skin rashes, diarrhoea or constipation, mood swings, irritability, hyperactivity and sometimes learning difficulties. Allergic reactions may be mistaken for recurrent colds or digestive upsets.

Extreme allergic reactions to a particular food, such as shellfish, peanuts and strawberries, are relatively rare. The face, mouth and throat may become swollen and create breathing difficulties. This requires urgent medical treatment.

Allergies have become increasingly common in the last decade, for reasons yet to be clarified. Many natural therapists feel that escalating exposure to pollutants is partly to blame. Certain manmade chemicals such as pesticides are known to alter the functioning of the immune system. Although yet to be proven, some suspect that childhood vaccinations may also have something to do with the rising incidence of allergies in children.

Allergic symptoms are usually managed by reducing exposure to the offending substances. As many allergens such as grass pollen and dust are difficult to eliminate totally, complementary medicine places greater emphasis on strengthening the body's natural resistance. This enhances sufferers' tolerance to irritants and may actually free them from their symptoms altogether.

Diet and Nutritional Therapy

Prevention is far easier than cure. If allergies run in the family, it is best to breastfeed your baby for as long as possible. Research suggests that breastfed babies are far less likely to suffer from allergies than those given formula milk.

A wholesome diet supplying all the essential nutrients plays a vital role in the management of allergies.

Many allergy sufferers improve when they follow the naturopathic diet:

* plenty of fresh fruits and vegetables
* red meat no more than once or twice a week
* no dairy products
* no processed foods containing artificial additives or colourings
* plenty of mineral water (at least 6 glasses a day).

Those suffering from allergies often have low levels of certain nutrients, especially the B vitamins pantothenic acid (B_5) and pyridoxine (B_6), along with the minerals calcium, zinc and magnesium. These deficiencies can be corrected and prevented by giving a multi-vitamin and mineral supplement daily.

Vitamins A (as beta carotene) and E play a role in maintaining healthy mucus membranes, which are the body's first line of defence against allergens. These nutrients can be found in green leafy vegetables, carrots, apricots, wheatgerm and cold-pressed vegetable oils.

Vitamin C can neutralize histamine and so help to reduce allergic reactions. Give 500 mg (250 mg for under-threes) of vitamin C at the first sign of symptoms; repeat this dose up to 3 times a day until symptoms have cleared.

Relaxation

Stress has a disruptive influence on the immune system and allergies are often precipitated and exacerbated during times of emotional upheaval. Finding ways to help your child relax and unwind often helps with allergic troubles.

Professional Therapy

Homoeopathy

While there are many remedies that can treat the acute symptoms of allergies, homoeopathy is most effective when a constitutional remedy is given to boost general health and resilience to allergens. Consult a qualified homoeopath for more information.

Doctor's Prescription

Skin-patch testing can help to identify specific allergens. As it is not always possible to avoid an offending substance, sodium cromoglycate and steroid nasal sprays may be prescribed to 'dampen down' the allergic reaction when symptoms are severe.

See also **Asthma, Eczema, Food Allergies, Hay Fever, Hives**

ANXIETY

A state of worrying about anything and everything. The mind is constantly occupied with anxious thoughts. This psychological stress spills over into the body.

Typical Symptoms

Tight breathing, palpitations, loss of appetite, digestive upsets, sleeplessness and a variety of other non-specific ailments. Anxious children are often withdrawn and non-communicative or clingy and insecure. Anxiety can also aggravate allergic conditions such as **Asthma**, **Eczema** and **Hay Fever**.

Children probably suffer from anxiety more than we realize. Beginning nursery, changing school routines, being unwell, parental squabbles, starting potty training and generally being over-stimulated by well-meaning parents can all make a child anxious.

Babies seem to go through anxious phases, too, at which times they are particularly clingy and burst into tears as soon as you walk out of the room. This may be because they are teething, have an upset stomach or are feeling under the weather.

There is also a phenomenon known as separation anxiety which may explain why a baby is fretful. Some psychologists postulate that until the age of 4 to 6 months a baby is so close and dependent on his mother that he may not even realize he is separate from her. Separation anxiety comes from the awareness that he is indeed an independent person. It is therefore natural to be anxious about losing the person you love and depend upon to look after you.

At this stage unfamiliar situations and people can seem very frightening without mother or father there to give reassurance and protection. A baby also has no concept of time, so that being left with someone else for even just a few hours may seem like an eternity.

During this phase, which may last many months, it is probably best to make baby feel as secure as you can. Do not take any notice of those who say you will 'spoil' your baby or make a rod for your own back. A happy baby is one who feels safe and secure.

Aromatherapy and Massage

Touch works wonders for any anxiety condition. A soothing foot massage is a particularly effective way to comfort a fretful baby.

Working both feet at the same time, rub with your thumbs from the centre of the sole of the foot, over the ball and towards the bottom of the toes. Repeat until baby is settled.

You can either do this though baby's clothes or use the following aromatherapy oils:

* Chamomile and Lavender are particularly soothing; both are safe to use on newborn babies. Add the appropriate number of drops of either essence (*see page 6*) to an Almond oil base. This aromatherapy oil can be used to massage the feet or can be added to the bath.

* For children over 6: a 50:50 blend of Chamomile and Lavender can be dropped onto the pillow and used in a vaporizer to fragrance the bedroom.

Flower Remedies

* Emergency Essence (Jan de Vries) – a soothing blend of Chamomile, Lavender, Red Clover, Purple Coneflower, Self-Heal and Yarrow flower essences to ease all kinds of emotional upset.

* White Chestnut (Bach Flower Remedies, Healing Herbs) – for persistent unwanted thoughts, restless mental chatter, confusion, nervous worry, insomnia and headaches.

Diet and Nutritional Therapy

Anxiety states are related to a lack of certain nutrients, specifically vitamins B_1 and B_6, as well as the minerals calcium and magnesium.

An anxious child needs a wholesome, well-balanced diet with the emphasis on foods rich in these nutrients. A broad-spectrum vitamin and mineral supplement can be given for a month to see if there is any improvement in temperament, but it is not wise to give any of the vitamins or minerals singly as they can upset the balance of others in the body.

Other Helpful Remedies

Herbal Remedies

* Make an infusion from a blend of Chamomile flowers, Lime flowers and Orange blossom. Add 1 teaspoon of each herb to a pint (600 ml) of boiling water. When cooled, give the recommended dosage (*see page 30*). Avoid giving any drinks containing caffeine, such as cocoa, cola, coffee or tea, as this stimulating chemical can make your child feel more anxious.

* Children's Stress Formula (*see page 32*): 10 drops in 6 fl oz/180 ml of water 2 to 3 times a day.

Biochemic Tissue Salts

* Kali phos is particularly good for babies. Give 2 tablets 3 times a day.

Reflexology

Apply gentle reflex pressure to the solar plexus, adrenal gland and pancreas reflex areas on the feet and hands (*see Figure 2, page 53*).

Professional Therapy

Homoeopathy

A professional will consider anxiety as part of a whole symptom profile.

Doctor's Prescription

Anxiety is generally considered to be a transient problem. As children react to any inherent anxiety in either parent, the well-being of both mother and father should be considered. Doctors and health visitors can offer advice and support.

APPETITE PROBLEMS *See* **Feeding Problems**

ASTHMA

Asthma is the most common chronic childhood illness and has become even more prevalent and severe in recent years. It is now thought that 1 in 7 children living in Britain suffers from asthma to one degree or another. According to the World Health Organization, the same trend can be seen in most developed countries.

Typical Symptoms

Anything from a dry cough (particularly at night) and wheezing to a full-blown attack which leaves the sufferer fighting for breath. A tight feeling creeps across the chest, and the muscles in the airways go into spasm, making each breath a struggle. Panic often sets in making the heart race and intensifying the symptoms. Some children have only one of these symptoms, usually a persistent cough.

In asthmatics the tiny airways or bronchioles are, to some extent, constantly inflamed, making them especially sensitive to certain things that are inhaled. Symptoms occur when the bronchioles become swollen and irritated, usually in response to breathing in an allergen. This blocks the airflow to the tiny air sacs (alveoli) at the end of the bronchioles. Irritation stimulates the muscles around the bronchioles to tighten or constrict, reducing the airflow even more. These changes cause the typical symptoms of asthma.

Asthma is more common and starts earlier in boys (from 3 years old) than girls (from 8 years old). If allergies such as hay fever run in the family, your child is more at risk of suffering from asthma. Babies who have recurrent colds and catarrh or eczema are increasingly likely to develop asthma.

Attacks are triggered by emotional upset and stressful situations. The asthmatic child is often highly strung, nervous and sensitive.

A child is only considered to be asthmatic if symptoms occur at least three times, several family members suffer from allergies and/or there is some other reason to suspect symptoms will recur.

Coughing and wheezing can also be caused by other health problems, for instance viral infections such as colds and bronchitis, and genetic lung diseases such as cystic fibrosis. X-rays, blood tests and lung function tests may be necessary to make a correct diagnosis.

It is essential for your child to be diagnosed by a health professional and for his symptoms to be carefully monitored. Asthma attacks can be life-threatening and there are times when medication is essential. Self-help remedies can work alongside orthodox drugs, helping to reduce the frequency and severity of attacks.

Common Triggers for Asthma

* cigarette smoke – if the mother smokes during pregnancy this affects her baby's lung development and increases the risk of the child having asthma later

* air pollution – not just car exhaust fumes outdoors but moulds, house dust, dust mites, animal dander, feather pillows and duvets indoors
* grass, flower and tree pollens – provoke asthma attacks and seasonal allergies in some children
* exercise – especially in cold, dry air, triggers symptoms in 90 per cent of asthmatics
* food additives – especially yellow dyes, sodium benzoate and sulphites
* colds – cold viruses trigger wheezing in 80 to 85 per cent of asthmatic children
* emotional stress
* aspirin – the most common medication causing asthma flare-ups
* perfumes – in hair sprays, deodorants, furniture polish, etc.

Pinpointing Asthma Triggers

Keep a diary and write down everything that affects your child – record when attacks occur and their severity, then look for a pattern to emerge. Once you have established the key triggers, try to minimize your child's exposure to them as much as possible.

Practical Advice

Keep your child's bedroom as clean as possible. At least once a week, dust with a damp cloth and vacuum thoroughly. Keep fluffy toys away from your child, especially during the night. Limit your child to one or two favourite toys, and wash these regularly to remove dust.

Steam-cleaning carpets and mattresses on a regular basis may be helpful. Experts at Glasgow University claim superheated steam destroys dust mites and the allergens contained in their droppings.

Consider changing feather pillows and duvets for non-allergic varieties. Wash sheets, pillow cases and blankets weekly in hot water to kill dust mites.

Free-standing electronic air filters can help to remove airborne asthma triggers inside the home.

As mould spores are common asthma-provokers it is a good idea to keep the humidity in your home to less than 50 per cent.

Do not allow furry pets to sleep in your child's bedroom.

Diet and Nutritional Therapy

* Make sure your child drinks plenty of pure spring water. Fluids help to keep mucus secretions thin and loose, preventing them from becoming dry, sticky and difficult to clear from the lungs.

* Low dietary magnesium intake is associated with increased wheezing. Good dietary sources of magnesium are wholegrains, soya beans, nuts, shrimp and green leafy vegetables.

* The oils from fatty fish such as mackerel, salmon, sardines and tuna may reduce the body's production of inflammatory chemicals. Include these types of fish in your child's diet, or consider giving fish oil supplements.

* Onions, asparagus, turnips, cabbage and Brussels sprouts appear to be beneficial for all kinds of respiratory disorders including asthma.

* Studies have shown that giving vitamin B_6 supplements can produce a noticeable reduction in the frequency and severity of symptoms. As the dosages required are high, this should only be done under the supervision of a qualified nutritionist to ensure there is no danger of over-dosing.

* Try the following fresh juice blend: 4 oz/120 g of

raspberries, 4 oz/120 g strawberries and 1 orange. Give 5 fl oz/150 ml a day.

* Sunflower seeds are reputedly beneficial for asthmatics and the flowers are traditionally used to treat many types of chest problems. Sprinkle ground up seeds over natural yoghurt and honey, and into breakfast cereals.

Relaxation

Asthma attacks can be triggered by emotional upset and stressful events. Asthma symptoms are also stressful. Many sufferers panic about not being able to breathe properly, which exacerbates symptoms further.

Relaxation can play an important role in preventing attacks and keeping them from spiralling out of control.

Teaching your child a basic form of stress management, such as a simple meditation technique, will be valuable for the rest of his life.

Massage works wonders for relieving stress. Try to give your child a regular body massage at least once a week. On a daily basis, massage perhaps just the feet, hands or shoulders.

Using Lavender or Geranium in a carrier of Sunflower oil, massage the back using long sweeping movements. Start at the base of the spine, placing your hands on either side of the vertebrae, then sweep up the back, over the shoulders and down the sides of the body.

For children over 7 years old you can also use Cypress and Frankincense together or blended with one of the other essences mentioned here (e.g, Lavender with Cypress, or Geranium with Frankincense).

Other Helpful Remedies

Aromatherapy

* Spray your child's mattress with dilute Lavender or

Tea Tree essence (2 drops to 1/2 pint/300 ml) when changing the bedding. This will help to kill dust mites.

Homoeopathy

* Aconite if symptoms come on suddenly in the late evening or night and are accompanied by anxiety; worse for cold weather. Give 1 dose of the 6C potency every hour for up to 3 doses. Give another 2–3 doses if required and there has been some improvement after the initial dose. Consult a professional homoeopath if home prescribing brings no relief from symptoms.

Herbal Remedies

* A soothing tisane of Hyssop (made from the flowers and green tops) can help to clear the lungs.

* You could also try a little Lobelia tincture.

Naturopathy

Yoga breathing methods strengthen the lungs and diaphragm. Get your child to place his hands on his abdomen and breathe in slowly, feeling his stomach pushing out. Ask him to hold this for a moment, then breathe out slowly.

Plunging the feet into a hot foot bath can help to ease an attack.

Reflexology

Try massaging the reflex area between the big toe and second toe on both feet (*see Figure 2, page 53*).

Chinese Medicine

Professional treatment works to rebalance the whole meridian system, as the lung and bladder meridians are often blocked or congested in asthma sufferers. Acupuncture or acupressure and a personally prescribed blend of herbs can help.

* A traditional home remedy is Ma Huang – a warming herb that relaxes the lungs – and Chinese Liquorice, which helps to clear away mucus. Add 5 drops of each tincture to 1 cup (240 ml) of boiling water. Give as sips when tepid.

* Try working the Kidney 27 acupressure point – *see Figure 1, page 13*.

Professional Therapy

Osteopathy

The Osteopathic Centre for Children (London) treats many asthmatic children successfully. While a tendency to suffer from asthma can run in families, it can be a physical trauma that triggers the first attack. A severe blow to the back, for instance, may produce tension in the area of the chest and diaphragm; this in turn sets the scene for breathing problems. Treatments are aimed at relieving any residual tension and restoring a sense of balance.

Homoeopathy

There are 280 remedies that could be prescribed for asthma. While various homoeopathic remedies will help to relieve acute symptoms, a professional homoeopath will initially prescribe a constitutional remedy to strengthen the body's natural resistance to allergy triggers.

Doctor's Prescription

Medical treatment consists of an inhaled beta-agonist such as Ventolin (salbutamol) to relax the airways, and inhaled steroids such as Becotide (beclomethasome) to reverse inflammation and reduce swelling in the airways. Inhaled steroids are the mainstay of asthma treatment. They shorten the duration of acute asthma, help to prevent its onset and protect against long-term lung damage. Their effect on growth is minimal. During a more severe attack, oral steroids (Prednisolone) are given for 7 to 14 days. They should not cause harmful side-effects when used for such a short time.

Drug therapy may only have to be a short-term measure, as many infants grow out of their asthma.

Seek immediate help if your child is struggling to breathe as a result of an asthma attack.

See also **Allergies**, **Bronchitis and Bronchiolitis**, **Colds**, **Hay Fever**

ATHLETE'S FOOT

A fungal infection of the skin usually found between the toes which can affect children as well as adults. Athlete's foot can be caught by walking barefoot where someone with the infection has been. Swimming pools are common breeding grounds for this infectious fungus.

Fungal infections are more likely to appear when the immunity is low such as after an illness and at times of stress. Taking antibiotics, which kill off the beneficial bacteria that help to keep fungi in check, can create the right conditions for getting athlete's foot.

Typical Symptoms

White skin between the toes which is spongy or flaky, itchy or sore.

Prevention

Fungi thrive in dark, damp places, so keep the feet clean and dry.

Natural fibres should be worn close to the skin (cotton socks and leather shoes). Allow your child to go barefoot as much as possible. Do not let your child share or borrow shoes or socks.

Diet and Nutritional Therapy

* Strengthening the immune system is the best way to clear up athlete's foot and keep it away.
* Encourage your child to eat plenty of lightly cooked vegetables, wholegrain cereals, fish and lean meat.
* Limit all sugary foods such as biscuits, cakes, sweets, dried fruits, honey and sweet drinks such as squashes. Fruit juices (apple or orange, for example) are fine once or twice a day but should be diluted 50:50 with spring water.
* Garlic has anti-fungal properties, so use it abundantly in cooking – some children enjoy the taste of garlic, but if not, try giving garlic capsules instead.

Hydrotherapy and Herbs

* Bathe feet regularly in an infusion of Marigold flowers. You could also add 10 drops of Marigold tincture and 10 drops of Myrrh tincture to a footbath. Your child should soak his feet for at least 5 minutes once a day.
* Dry between the toes thoroughly with a towel and dust with Calendula (Marigold) talcum powder. If skin is dry and cracked, use Calendula cream instead.

Other Helpful Remedies

Aromatherapy

* Tea Tree has potent anti-fungal properties. Make a therapeutic footbath by placing a handful of coarse

sea salt into a bowl of warm water and add 5 drops of Tea Tree essence. The feet should be soaked in this way for 5 minutes a day until the condition clears.

* For babies over 6 months old: Add Tea Tree essence to the bath, then massage the affected area with the essential oil in a base of Almond oil. Afterwards allow your child to go barefoot *(see page 6 for appropriate amount of drops)*.
* Natural athlete's foot powder: Add 10 drops of Tea Tree essence to 1 cup (240 ml) of dry, green clay or talc (available from most healthfood shops). Mix really well and powder the feet with this each day.

Doctor's Prescription

Anti-fungal powders and creams are available without a prescription. If the toenails are involved, your doctor may prescribe oral anti-fungal agents or an anti-fungal nail varnish.

B

BEDWETTING

Around 10 per cent of children still wet their bed during the night at the age of 5; some continue for several years afterwards.

Bedwetting, or *enuresis* as it is known medically, is usually a sign that the part of the brain that controls urination is slow to mature, so it is best not to worry unduly because your child will grow out of it. Perhaps you have tried to start potty training before your child is really ready to be out of nappies at night.

If your child is over 6 years old, bedwetting might be due to an emotional or psychological problem. The birth of a brother or sister, moving house, changing schools or family stresses are possible reasons why your child may be anxious, worried or feeling insecure. Wetting the bed could also be your child's way of getting some attention if he feels he has not seen enough of you during the day.

Sometimes bedwetting is a caused by a physical problem such as cystitis or a urinary tract infection. Typical signs of this are frequent urination with a burning sensation. If accidents occur during the day too, there may be an anatomical abnormality of the kidneys.

Practical Advice

Try to discover whether your child is worried; if so, offer plenty of reassurance. If he wets the bed, change the sheets swiftly without making a fuss. Leave clean bedding and clothes out for older children so they can change themselves with a minimum of fuss.

Homoeopathy

Several different homoeopathic remedies may be helpful; try to choose the one which best matches your child's symptoms:

* Causticum – for bedwetting that occurs during the first sleep. There may be involuntary loss of urine in the day if over-excited or while coughing or sneezing. Your child will be anxious, fearful at night, irritable and tearful over the tiniest things.
* Pulsatilla – for the child who is fearful at twilight, anxious at night, capricious, changeable, clingy.
* Sepia – wets the bed in the first part of sleep, weepy and prefers to be alone. (More common among girls.)

Give the 30C potency, 1 tablet each day for up to 3 days. If there is improvement, repeat each week until the bedwetting ceases.

If the bedwetting persists, consult a professional homoeopath.

Flower Remedies

Flower remedies are particularly helpful when there is a strong psychological element in bedwetting.

* Cherry Plum (Bach Flower Remedies, Healing Herbs) – for feeling unable to control thoughts and emotions, impulses of losing control, obsessive fears
* Crab Apple (Bach Flower Remedies, Healing Herbs) – for those who feel unclean, leading to feelings of despondency and self-disgust

* Dog Rose (Australian Bush Flower Remedies) – for fearful, shy children who are apprehensive of others and have niggling fears

* Surfgrass (Pacific Essences) – for courage and strength, with a beneficial effect on the kidneys.

Give 2 drops 3 times a day until the condition improves.

Other Helpful Remedies

Naturopathy

Avoid foods or drinks containing stimulants or diuretics, such as cola drinks, as well as white sugar and food colourings, especially orange.

Aromatherapy

* Add Chamomile or Lavender to your child's night-time bath. You could also massage the lower back with the same essence in a carrier of Almond oil before bedtime, or use Hypericum (St John's Wort) macerated oil.

Herbal Remedy

* Make an infusion of Chamomile, Marshmallow Root or St John's Wort. Give the recommended dose (*see page 30*) warm and sweetened with honey to taste. Cornsilk tisane is particularly effective at soothing irritation, often responsible for bedwetting in older children.

Chinese Medicine

* Add ginger and walnuts to the diet. Use ground ginger in gingerbread, biscuits and milk-puddings. Sprinkle ground ginger onto fruit, and ground walnuts onto yoghurt and cereals.

Reflexology

Massage the bladder reflex area on the base of the feet and between the thumb and wrist (*see Figure 2, page 53*) each night for 2 minutes.

Professional Therapy

Osteopathy

May be recommended as there may be residual tension in the pelvic area which needs to be released.

Doctor's Prescription

Drug therapy uses anti-diuretic hormones which suppress the urge to urinate, or Tofranil (an anti-depressant), but the problem may return when therapy is discontinued. Behaviour therapy may be used, for example star charts or alarms which sound when the mattress is wet.

BEHAVIOURAL PROBLEMS

Even easy-going, compliant and gentle children are not going to be little angels all the time. There is a whole range of undesirable behaviour which is completely natural and normal in children, so what is seen as 'difficult' has to be considered in context.

When a child is growing up, he is constantly pushing out on all fronts and experimenting with different types of behaviour. Some children are aware of 'naughtiness' at an early age, but are not mature enough to control this behaviour. What you do to contain your child's behaviour can either ameliorate or exacerbate the situation.

There is no doubt that children need boundaries. They need to know very clearly what is and what is not acceptable to you. Be as consistent as possible, otherwise your child may become confused. Allowing one kind of behaviour at home and expecting another when visiting Granny is not going to work.

Children are also more likely to misbehave when they are tired, bored, hungry or threatening for an illness – something worth bearing in mind when formulating your response.

Clear instructions and praise invariably work better than nagging, criticism and chastisement.

Practical Advice

* Use rewards or incentives to teach your child how you want him to behave.
* Separate the behaviour from the child; if you constantly tell a child that he is bad, he may become that way.
* Avoid situations which invite misbehaviour, such as going shopping when your child is tired or hungry.
* Try to make events he does not like, such as hair washing, into a game rather than going into battle over it.
* Punishment does not teach your child how you want him to behave, only how you don't. Children are mimics: if you want them to act in a certain way, set a good example.

Diet and Nutritional Therapy

Difficult behaviour may be linked to a food allergy, specific nutritional deficiencies, excessive refined carbohydrates and sugary foods, food colourings (especially red and orange) and preservatives.

If diet is implicated in your child's difficult behaviour, other signs might be a constant stuffy or runny nose, frequent infections such as colds, coughs and ear infections, abdominal bloating, constipation or diarrhoea and episodes of inappropriate fatigue. He may also have cravings for sweets, chocolates or sugary foods and an excessive thirst.

As a preventative measure follow the basic naturopathic diet (*see page 48*) and stay away from all processed and coloured foods.

A good breakfast is essential, and mealtimes should be as regular as possible. Children tend to be more cranky, disobedient and likely to have tantrums if they have skipped a meal, and often settle down when given something to eat, provided it is wholesome and nutritious.

Other Helpful Therapies

Herbal Remedy

* Happy Child Formula (*see page 33*) can be helpful. Give 10 drops in 6 fl oz/180 ml of cooled boiled water 3 times a day.

Professional Therapies

Nutrition

To pinpoint and correct food allergies or nutritional deficiencies it is essential to consult a qualified nutritionist.

Homoeopathy

Can help with a whole spectrum of behavioural problems from hyperactivity to jealousy of a newborn sibling. Consult a professional homoeopath.

Doctor's Prescription

Very difficult or upsetting behaviour may be referred to a child psychologist, who will see both child and parents together.

See also **Hyperactivity, Irritability, Moodiness, Temper Tantrums**

BITES AND STINGS

Insect bites vary from being itchy and irritating to red, swollen and painful. Most insects – including bees, wasps, mosquitoes and midges – only become a nuisance during the warmer months. Protecting children from being bitten is undoubtedly the best policy. In some countries insects also spread infection and disease; in these cases prevention is particularly important.

If your child is bitten by an animal, especially a wild one such as a mouse (brought in by the cat, for example), it is important to consult a doctor before using any of the natural remedies recommended to heal the injury.

Natural Protection

Mosquitoes are at their most active at dusk and during the evening. When out in the garden, make sure your child's arms and legs are well covered to reduce the chance of being bitten. Dress him in light-coloured clothes, as dark ones attract insects.

Whenever insects are a nuisance, use a natural insect repellent (*see page 87*) on exposed areas of the body.

Treatment

If your child is stung or bitten, there are ways to ease the pain and discomfort.

Wash insect bites straight away with soap and water.

Bees leave both their sting and a poison bag in the skin; both need to be removed. Ease the sting, with attached bag, out gently with a clean fingernail or a pair of tweezers, taking care not to puncture or squeeze the bag.

Discourage children from scratching bites, as this only makes them worse and can lead to infection. Some of the remedies listed below relieve itching.

Aromatherapy

* For babies over 1 year old: 3 drops of Eucalyptus oil in 1 cup (240 ml) of an infusion of Lavender flowers. Dab or spray onto the skin.

* Citronella is a very effective insect repellent, best used in a vaporizer rather than directly on skin.

* Lavender oil contains anti-venom properties and often acts as an antidote to the poison of bee stings.

* To make a soothing Sting Relief oil, blend 2 drops of Lavender with 2 drops of Tea Tree in 30 ml Almond oil. Dab onto stings with a cotton bud. This is safe for all children over 6 months old.

* For newborn babies, use 2 drops of Lavender in 30 ml Almond oil.

Herbal Remedies

* Make an infusion of Lavender or Rosemary, then dab onto skin with cotton wool. This is safe for babies over 6 months old.

* A bunch of fresh Basil herb will keep flies away.

Naturopathy

* For instant relief, apply a cold compress made from

crushed ice cubes wrapped up in flannel.

* Bee stings are acidic and can be neutralized by dabbing with cotton wool soaked in a solution of bicarbonate of soda and water (2 teaspoons to 1 cup/240 ml of water).
* Wasp stings are alkaline and can be neutralized by dabbing them with cotton wool soaked in cider vinegar or lemon juice.
* To relieve the itching of other insect bites (such as mosquito bites), dissolve 1 teaspoon of baking soda in 1 cup (240 ml) water, soak a cotton wool ball in the solution and bathe the bites.

Homoeopathy

* Apis mel is the number one remedy for bites and stings. To be effective, symptoms should generally fit the following picture: swelling, redness, burning or stinging pains, restlessness, lack of thirst; better for cold applications, worse for heat and between 4 and 6 p.m.
* Ledum – better for puncture wounds and bites from both animals and insects. Pains are tearing and throbbing. The area is swollen, blue and cold but feels hot to the sufferer. Better for cold applications; worse for heat.
* Vespa – a more specific remedy for wasp stings. Give 1 dose of the 30C potency immediately and 1 dose daily until the symptoms clear.
* Apply neat Hypericum (St John's Wort) tincture to bites and stings to soothe and help prevent infection.

Doctor's Prescription

Calamine lotion applied with cotton wool will soothe the skin and relieve itching. Anti-histamine drugs are recommended for an allergic reaction. Antibiotics may be prescribed for infected bites.

Seek immediate help if your child appears to have an allergic reaction to an insect bite or sting.

Allergies occur in a small percentage of children and are characterized by the body swelling up and laboured breathing.

If the sting is in the mouth or throat, rinse your child's mouth with iced water or give ice cubes to suck and seek medical help immediately.

BRONCHITIS AND BRONCHIOLITIS

Acute bronchitis is a condition involving inflammation and infection of the respiratory tract, in which the bronchioles (tiny air ways) become filled with mucus. Bronchiolitis is a term that describes the same condition in babies under 18 months old.

Typical Symptoms

Mild fever with a cough; breathing that is a little faster than normal. The chest feels raw and oppressed. In babies, breathing can become unerringly rapid and laboured. Sufferer feels restless, distressed and irritable.

Coughs and colds often start these conditions off in children, but they can be caused by many different viruses. Bronchitis is particularly common during the winter months.

If a baby has bronchiolitis, keep him warm and give as much comfort in the form of cuddles as possible to stop him crying.

Diet and Nutritional Therapy

* Try to include plenty of fresh fruits and vegetables into your child's diet. Use watercress and garlic in cooking, incorporating into thick vegetable soups and other dishes.

* Watercress is particularly recommended by phytotherapists for treating bronchitis. Garlic possess antibiotic properties and helps to loosen mucus.
* Add marjoram and oregano to dishes; these herbs help to relieve bronchitis.
* Give freshly squeezed lemon juice diluted with hot water and sweetened with honey.

Aromatherapy

Essential oils are helpful for treating bronchial congestion because of their anti-viral and anti-bacterial properties. They can be inhaled and massaged into the chest.

* Use Lavender or Chamomile essences in a vaporizer placed in the bedroom overnight. Gently rub your child's chest with your chosen essence diluted in a carrier of Almond oil.
* For babies and children over 6 months old: Tea Tree or Eucalyptus can also be used.

Other Helpful Remedies

Herbal Remedies

* Give warm tisanes of Elderflower and Peppermint sweetened with honey in the early stages to encourage perspiration.
* If a cough develops, try an infusion of the flowers and green tops of Hyssop.
* Give 1 teaspoon of Little Ones' Cough Syrup (*see page 31*) 3 times a day.

Chinese Medicine

* Astragalus (Huang Qi) is used to boost the immune system. Add 5 to 10 drops to 1 cup (240 ml) of boiling water and give as sips when tepid.
* Work the Kidney 27 acupressure point – *see Figure 1, page 13* – to revitalize the flow of *qi* to the chest and lungs.

Biochemic Tissue Salts

* Kali phos, 2 tablets 3 times a day.

Doctor's Prescription

Antibiotics are prescribed for bronchitis. Bronchiolitis is a viral infection, so supportive measures such as humidified air, inhaled Ventolin (salbutamol) are used. Sometimes babies can become quite ill with bronchiolitis and develop difficulty breathing. They will be admitted to hospital.

Seek immediate medical help if the condition does not subside in a few days with bedrest. Bronchitis can become serious if the inflammation spreads to cause bronchopneumonia.

BRUISES

Bruised skin turns purplish or blackish blue as a result of being bumped or knocked. This discolouration occurs when minute blood capillaries lying just under the skin are temporarily damaged.

Some children (and adults) seem to bruise more easily than others.

Naturopathy

* Wrap some ice cubes in a flannel (or frozen peas in a kitchen towel) and hold against the affected area. Spray the bruise with cold water (use the shower nozzle, atomizer or pump-action bottle) as soon as it appears, and each day until it fades away.
* Vitamin C and bioflavonoids can strengthen the tiny blood capillaries, making them more resilient to damage. These nutrients can be found in most fresh fruits and vegetables, particularly citrus fruits, purple/black fruits such as black grapes, blackberries and bilberries, green peppers and parsley.

Aromatherapy

* Lavender essence helps to reduce the inflammation and speed healing. Add 2 drops to 30 ml of Hypericum oil, as this also has soothing and pain-relieving properties.

* For babies over 1 year old: use Lavender or Geranium.

Other Helpful Remedies

Homoeopathy

* Soak a pad of lint or cotton wool in distilled Witch Hazel or diluted tincture of Arnica (2 teaspoonfuls to a tea-cupful of cold water) and bind the compress firmly, but not tightly, in place. Keep the pad moist with your chosen remedy until the tenderness has subsided.
* Arnica – give 1 dose of the 30C potency straight away, and once a day until the pain goes.

* Rub Arnica ointment into the bruise immediately, but only if the skin is not broken.

Flower Remedies

* Give 2 drops of Rescue Remedy (Bach Flower Remedies) or Five Flower Remedy (Healing Herbs) immediately, on the tongue or in a glass of spring water, then every hour until the pain and shock subside.

Doctor's Prescription

As bruising usually disappears in 1 to 2 weeks, medical treatment in not usually necessary. An unusual amount of bruising may, however, indicate a blood-clotting disorder.

BURNS

Burns and scalds are usually caused by heat, although they can also occur as a result of friction or intense cold. Certain chemicals such as bleach are also capable of burning the skin.

Never leave hot tea, coffee, kettles or cooking pans within children's reach.

Natural remedies are only recommended for treating minor burns and scalds. More serious ones should go straight to casualty.

Hydrotherapy

* For burns caused by heat, pour cold water over the affected area immediately. Chemical burns should be washed with cold running water for at least 5 minutes.

* You can also make a cold compress by adding ice cubes to a bowl of cold water; put 2 drops of neat Lavender essence on a clean flannel and wring it out in the water. This usually prevents blistering.

Herbal Remedies

* Juice from the Aloe Vera plant is renowned for its ability to treat minor burns. It soothes inflammation, relieves pain and encourages the regeneration of new tissue. Apply liberally with cotton wool, dab onto the burn or wrap a piece of gauze saturated with aloe juice around the affected area. You could also apply Aloe Vera gel.

* Hypericum (St John's Wort) promotes healing and prevents burns from becoming infected. Add 1 teaspoon of Hypericum tincture to 1 cup (240 ml) of cooled boiled water. Soak a pad of gauze in this lotion, apply to the burn and cover with lint and a bandage. Keep the gauze moistened with a few drops of lotion until the scab begins to form, after which the burn should be kept as dry as possible.

* Alternatively, apply Hypericum ointment to the burn and either cover with a light dressing or leave exposed.

Other Helpful Remedies

Aromatherapy

* Lavender essence can be used undiluted (this is the only instance when an essential oil can be used neat) to soothe, prevent infection and promote new tissue growth. It does not sting even when used neat and the fragrance will help to restore feelings of calm.

Homoeopathy

* Cantharis is the number one remedy for burns and scalds accompanied by stinging, smarting pains. Give

1 dose of the 30C potency immediately and for the next 2 or 3 days.

* Aconite may be taken to ease shock. Give 1 dose of the 6C potency immediately and every 30 minutes for up to 4 doses.

* Homoeopathic burn ointment can help, but only if the skin is not broken – Urtica urens for minor burns (redness), Calendula cream for more severe burns (blistering).

Doctor's Prescription

Burns covering a large area should be seen by a doctor immediately. Cold burns (such as frostbite) should also be referred straight to your GP.

C

CHICKEN POX

A highly infectious disease spread by the chicken pox or shingles virus. It is spread by contact with another child with chicken pox, especially if he is coughing and sneezing.

Young babies usually get a mild form of chicken pox; the younger they are, the milder it is. Some only have a couple of spots.

Incubation period: 14 to 16 days.

Infectious period: from the day before the rash appears until all the spots are dry.

Typical Symptoms

A rash of itchy red spots like blisters or raised swellings containing a clear fluid. Starts with a feeling of being vaguely unwell, with headache, mild fever and slight nausea. Spots usually appear first on the chest and back, then spread to the rest of the body, eventually drying into scabs which fall off. The spots will disappear after about 12 days.

Follow the general guidelines for **Childhood Diseases**; *see also* **Infections**.

Homoeopathy

* See Special Recipe for Childhood Diseases (*page 99*).
* Dab Calendula cream or Hypericum ointment onto spots.
* Bathe the eyes with Euphrasia tincture – 1 drop in an eye bath, if there are any spots inside the lids. You can also give 1 dose of Euphrasia 30C.

Aromatherapy

* Lavender and Chamomile can help to soothe the rash.
* Lukewarm baths also help to relieve the itching. Add 2 drops of Lavender to 1 cup (240 ml) bicarbonate of soda and sprinkle into the bath.

Other Helpful Remedies

Herbal Remedies

* Chickweed tea is soothing when dabbed onto the skin with cotton wool. A cupful could also be added to the bath.
* Give sips of Chamomile or St John's Wort tisane,
* Echinacea tincture will help to support the immune system.

Naturopathy

* Apply cool wet towels to soothe the rash.
* Dab dilute cider vinegar onto very itchy spots; 1 tablespoon to 1 pint/600 ml of water, or add 1 cup/240 ml of cider vinegar to the bath.

Professional Therapy

Homoeopathy

While it is generally considered to be better for a child to get the disease, a professional homoeopath can give Varicella 30C as a protective measure during an outbreak of chickenpox.

Doctor's Prescription

Chicken pox is generally not considered to be serious in childhood. Sometimes a chest infection may complicate the illness and, if suspected, it is best to consult your doctor.

Contact with pregnant women should be avoided. If this occurs the expectant mother should seek medical advice. Contact with adults who have not had chicken pox (or, in rare cases, even when they have) should also be avoided, as the disease can be quite serious in adults.

Seek help if the spots become infected, i.e. there is redness or swelling around them, or pus oozing from them, if the itching is unbearable and is not helped by the above self-help measures, or if the spots affect the eyes (not just the eyelids).

CHILDHOOD DISEASES

In the early years of life, babies and children are susceptible to a range of infectious diseases which include rubella (German measles), chicken pox, measles, mumps and whooping cough.

Most parents are apprehensive about caring for a child with any of these infectious illnesses. Although symptoms are mostly manageable, occasionally they can cause extreme discomfort and in very rare cases there may be complications such as encephalitis (inflammation of the brain). Such possibilities can make these diseases all the more alarming.

Traditionally, childhood illnesses were regarded as an opportunity to develop strength and resilience. Although unpleasant at the time, a child suffering from a bout of chickenpox emerges endowed (in all but very rare cases) with lifelong immunity from the illness.

Most natural therapists such as naturopaths, homoeopaths and osteopaths still uphold the view that childhood illnesses are not necessarily a bad thing. They suggest that, so long as a child is healthy and well-nourished, symptoms should be relatively mild and manageable. A child blessed with plenty of natural vitality will make a speedy recovery and bounce back to health with ease.

Even so, it is important to nurse a sick child through a childhood disease. This may seem obvious, but there is a growing tendency to give children antibiotics or painkillers and encourage them to carry on a normal life. When this happens a child's vitality is lowered and he may feel under par for several weeks after the illness. Children who are not given sufficient time to rest and recuperate are then more likely to go down with one illness after another.

You will need to prepare yourself for devoting at least a week to caring for a sick child. Looking after a child who is feeble, miserable, whingy and in distress can be incredibly draining, both emotionally and physically. Do try to find ways of sustaining your own vitality and maintaining a sense of calm at this time.

Incubation period: the time between catching the illness and becoming unwell.

Infectious period: the time during which your child can pass the illness on to someone else.

Practical Advice

Sleep and bedrest are some of the best natural remedies for childhood diseases. Bedrest may help to prevent a fever and enables available energy to be channelled into fending off the illness for a speedy recovery.

Cuddle and stay with your baby or young child while he sleeps if necessary. When ill, some babies need plenty of reassurance and will only drift off if mother or father is close. This can be a good opportunity to catch up on your own sleep, too.

If baby is particularly clingy during the day, you could try carrying him around in a sling if you have chores to do.

Offer plenty of fluids to a sick baby or child, especially if he is feverish. Give mineral water, diluted freshly squeezed juices (which are rich in vitamins and minerals) and warm herbal teas sweetened with honey.

If breastfeeding your baby, continue to do so on demand as this will provide comfort as well as nourishment.

Give small, easily digestible, nutritious meals whenever your child feels hungry. Simple dishes are yoghurt with honey, stewed fruits and vegetable soups. The demand for certain nutrients increases when the body is fighting an infection and levels need to be topped up (*see* **Infections**).

Keep a hot, feverish child cool and comfortable (*see* **Fever**). Do not take a baby or a child with a fever out and about.

Try to avoid over-stimulating a sick baby or child by having lots of visitors or taking him shopping. Reading books to him in bed is more restful than letting him watch television.

Unusual symptoms such as rashes and spots can be alarming for a small child. It is reassuring to be told that these symptoms will only last for a short while and that he will soon be back to his normal self again.

Children who are distressed and fearful of their illnesses may be calmed by giving flower essences such as Rescue Remedy (Bach Flower Remedies), Five Flower Remedy (Healing Herbs), First Aid Flower Essence (Findhorn Flower Essences) or Emergency Essence (Jan de Vries)

Do not worry unduly if your child regresses to babyish behaviour. This is often a first sign that he is not well and, although irritating, will disappear when he begins to recover. Try to be tolerant and indulge your child during this time.

Discourage your child from overdoing things during the convalescent stage of an illness. Relapses are common at this vulnerable time.

For more specific remedies, see the suggestions for individual illnesses.

Homoeopathy

Annette Middleton has devised a special recipe of remedies for relieving the typical symptoms of chickenpox, measles, German measles and other 'spotty' illnesses.

Recipe for Spotty Illnesses

* Aconite 30c – at the first sign of a fever or other symptoms.
* Ant tart 30c – to help heal spots without scarring. Give 1 dose daily when the spots appear.
* Merc sol 30C – helps to bring out all the spots. Give 1 dose only.
* Rhus tox 30c – for feverish, extremely restless children with a very itchy rash. Give once or twice daily

for up to 10 days.
* Pulsatilla 30C – for the cough which often develops with these illnesses. Give 1 dose.
* Echinacea 30C – for spots around the eyes.

Herbal Remedies

* Children's Immunity Formula (*see page 32*) can be given as a preventative measure or to aid recovery.
* Give sips of Catnip tea sweetened with honey.

COELIAC DISEASE

Young children are the most likely sufferers of coeliac disease, for it usually strikes before the age of 3.

Typical Symptoms

Diarrhoea, with soft foul-smelling stools and sometimes a stomach swollen with wind.

Coeliac disease is characterized by an inability to digest or absorb food because of a sensitivity to gluten, a protein found in wheat, rye and other grains.

Why some children are unable to absorb gluten remains a mystery, but the disease tends to run in families and sometimes occurs after a bowel infection.

Some believe coeliac disease may be related to weaning infants onto cereals too early. They recommend breastfeeding until baby is at least 4 months old, then limiting cereal intake to baby rice and millet for at least the first year.

If you think your child may be suffering from coeliac disease, it is essential to consult your doctor before embarking on any of the following recommendations.

Diet and Nutritional Therapy

* All foods containing gluten need to be removed from the diet. This means excluding all grains except for brown rice, millet and corn. This includes foods such as bread, cakes, biscuits, processed foods in general, and any food cooked or thickened with flour or covered in batter or bread crumbs.
* Milk can also upset some coeliac sufferers.
* A wholesome gluten-free diet comprises fresh vegetables including potatoes, brown rice, plain fish, dried beans, fruit, cheese, cream, eggs, bacon, fresh meat, honey and full-fruit jam.
* Vitamin and mineral deficiencies may result from the inability to digest and absorb nutrients properly. Calcium levels are often low in those suffering from coeliac disease. A qualified nutritionist can help to identify specific nutrients that may need topping up. It may be a good idea to give a broad spectrum multi-vitamin and mineral supplement to ensure your child gets sufficient quantities on a daily basis.

Herbal Remedies

Some herbs are particularly soothing to the mucous membranes lining the stomach and intestines.

* Marshmallow Root – make an infusion, strain and give the appropriate dosage (*see page 30*).
* Slippery Elm – give $1/2$ – 1 teaspoon of the ground powder in warm water twice a day.

Many herbalists feel there is a link between coeliac disease and bottle-feeding babies. The treatment prescribed aims to restore the imbalance of beneficial micro-organisms in the gut and strengthen the immune system, using herbs appropriate to each individual.

Doctor's Prescription

Diagnosis of coeliac disease can involve taking a small sample (biopsy) of the gut for examination and blood tests. A gluten-free diet is necessary; products such as gluten-free flour, biscuits and pasta can be prescribed by your doctor. The condition may improve spontaneously.

COLDS

Colds are caused by hundreds of different cold viruses. Babies are particularly susceptible because they have yet to build up immunity to the many viruses in circulation. Breastfeeding gives babies a degree of protection, especially if mother already has some resistance to a particular cold virus.

Children often get one cold after another when they first start nursery or playschool, as they are constantly coming into contact with different strains of virus.

Natural remedies can be very effective at keeping colds at bay as well as relieving their symptoms.

Typical Symptoms

Bouts of sneezing and a blocked or runny nose are tell-tale signs of a developing cold. A sore throat, headache, dry tickly cough and general washed-out feeling add to the misery of a typical cold.

Babies cannot blow their noses, so breathing and feeding can be difficult.

Diet and Nutritional Therapy

* Vitamin C is renowned for its ability to ward off colds. At the very first sign of symptoms, give vitamin C with bioflavonoids to enhance absorption (500 mg 3 times a day for children over 3 years old; 250 mg for those under 3). If you are breastfeeding, increase your own intake of vitamin C (1 g 3 times a day).
* The following vitamin C-rich fresh juice blend can be helpful: 1 grapefruit, 1 orange and 4 oz/120g of strawberries. Give 5 fl oz/150 ml daily.
* The mineral zinc plays an important role in maintaining a healthy and efficient immune system. New research from a New York university suggests that zinc supplementation can reduce the time-span of a cold by half and, if taken early enough, can stop a cold very quickly. The best way to take zinc for colds is in the form of suckable lozenges.

Aromatherapy

Essential oils can protect babies and children from colds as well as relieve symptoms.

* Peppermint and Eucalyptus – blend the appropriate number of drops of either (*see page 6*) in a base of Almond oil and massage into the chest and back. To benefit from the vapours, add the essences to the bath and use in a vaporizer in your child's bedroom overnight.
* For babies under 6 months: Eucalyptus only. Try adding 3 drops of essence to a small bowl of boiling water and place under baby's cot at night.
* For children over 5: Black Pepper or Rosemary can also be used.

* Steam inhalation helps to relieve congestion in the nose and chest. Add 2 drops of essence to a basin of steaming hot water; cover your child's head with a towel and encourage slow, deep breathing. Always supervise steam inhalations.
* You can to some extent protect babies and children from catching someone else's cold by making a solution using 2 drops Peppermint and 2 drops Eucalyptus in $1/_2$ pint (300 ml) of water. Spray this around the house.

Other Helpful Remedies

Herbal Remedies

* Echinacea helps to prevent and relieve colds by strengthening the body's immune defences. Add 5 to 10 drops of Echinacea tincture to warm water, fruit juice or milk, depending on preference. Give 3 times a day.
* You could also give the Children's Immunity Formula (*see page 32*): 10 drops in 6 fl oz/180 ml cooled boiled water 3 times a day.
* Alternatively you could give Elderflower Syrup (*see page 31*).
* When the first symptoms appear, try giving your child a warm tisane of Lemon Balm and Chamomile flowers sweetened with honey.
* Garlic is a natural antibiotic which helps to combat colds. During the winter, give 1 to 2 capsules a day as a preventative measure. Many children like the taste of garlic, so use liberally in cooking.

Homoeopathy

* Aconite can help to nip colds in the bud.
* Ferrum phos may be better if the cold starts with a sore throat.

Give the 6C potency every 2 hours for up to 4 doses during the early stages of a cold.

There are many possible remedies for colds depending on the profile of symptoms; the following ones are among the most helpful:

* Allium cepa – when there is lots of sneezing, streaming nose and eyes
* Pulsatilla – for babies and children who have thick, creamy catarrh and want to be cuddled all the time
* Sambucus nigra – for snuffles in newborn babies

Give 1 dose of the 6C potency 3 times a day for 2 to 3 days.

If your child suffers from recurrent colds, it is best to consult a professional homoeopath who can prescribe a constitutional remedy for strengthening his natural resistance.

Dietary Therapy

Apple and cinnamon tea can help to soothe cold symptoms. Cut a whole apple into chunks and boil for 20 minutes with a stick of cinnamon, then strain and give to drink when still warm, sweetened with honey.

Chinese Medicine

* Warming ginger tea soothes a sore throat and eases congestion. Add 1 teaspoon of fresh grated ginger root to 1 cup (240 ml) of boiling water, allow to steep for 5 minutes, strain and add 1 teaspoon of brown

sugar. Give your child sips of this drink throughout the day.

Reflexology

Massage the reflex points for the head and lungs on the feet and hands (*see Figure 2, page 53*). To enhance the benefits of the massage, use an aromatherapy oil.

Biochemic Tissue Salts

* Nat mur: 2 tablets 3 times a day.

Doctor's Prescription

As colds are caused by viruses, symptoms such as a blocked nose will not be helped by antibiotics. A persistently blocked nose should be checked out as it may be due to enlarged adenoids.

Seek help if cold symptoms have not begun to clear after a week. Colds can be forerunners of something more serious, so if your baby or child has a temperature, is feverish, is off his food and cries inconsolably, consult your doctor.

COLIC

Colic usually occurs for the first time in the third or fourth week of life; it can be a distressing time for parents as well as babies. Fortunately most infants outgrow colic by the time they are 3 or 4 months old.

No one knows exactly what causes colic and why it should affect some babies and not others. Some suggest that a baby's immature digestive system has difficulty processing food, which leads to a form of indigestion. The undigested food is then fermented by intestinal bacteria which produce the air bubbles responsible for the pain and distension of colic.

Colic is generally worse in the evenings, often coming on at around 6 p.m. It can last for several hours.

Relief often comes after burping, passing wind or filling a nappy. You may notice the stool is slightly greenish in colour.

Typical Symptoms

Sharp, intermittent stomach pains or cramps. A baby with colic cries or screams and is difficult to console by holding, cuddling or gently rocking. Baby may draw his legs up or stretch them out rigidly.

Practical Advice

Some babies swallow air with their feeds, which may cause colic if they cannot bring it up easily. This can happen in breastfed babies when the milk flow is too strong, as well as bottlefed babies if the teat is too big (for new babies) or too small (for older ones). Experiment with different feeding positions or a teat with a different-sized hole.

Try to prevent your baby becoming desperate for food, as he will gulp down air when crying and when sucking too frantically.

Always sit baby upright after feeds and rub his back to bring up wind. This is worthwhile even if baby has dropped off to sleep, as he will soon drift off again and is more likely to sleep soundly as a result.

Try to relax when breastfeeding a colicky baby. The nervous tension of an anxious mother can upset an infant enough to interfere with his digestion.

It is natural to want to nurse a crying baby, but as a colicky baby is not digesting properly, extra milk may only aggravate the problem when all baby really wants is a comfort suck. Offering your finger, a dummy or a bottle of tepid water can often ease baby's distress more effectively.

Colicky babies are often soothed by being carried around upright in a baby sling – also worth a try if you have chores to do around the house.

Naturopathy

If you are breastfeeding baby it is important to eat a good balanced diet with plenty of fruit and vegetables and to drink plenty of pure mineral water.

It is possible that you are eating something that is causing the colic. If you have a food allergy or an intolerance to certain foods, be sure to exclude these from your diet. Cow's milk is a common culprit, so cutting out dairy produce for a few days and seeing if this brings relief may be worth a try.

Other foods which may provoke colic in breastfed babies are:

* Caffeine (in tea, coffee and cola drinks), chocolate; citrus fruits (grapefruit, orange and lemons), strawberries, grapes; garlic, onions, green peppers, broccoli and cauliflower. Hot spicy food can also cause problems so it is best to avoid such dishes.

* Some bottlefed babies are allergic to cow's milk which can cause colicky pains, diarrhoea or constipation. These babies often fare much better when given a soya formula instead.

* If baby is weaned, avoid bananas, yoghurt, lettuce and 'gassy' foods such as beans and turnips.

Aromatherapy and Massage

* Colic can often be helped by massaging baby's tummy gently. Lie baby on his back and gently rub his abdomen in a clockwise direction using two or three of your fingers. If your baby prefers to be on his tummy, place

him across your lap and gently rub back and forth across his lower back.

* The benefits can be enhanced by using an aromatherapy massage oil: 2 drops Fennel or 2 drops Dill to 30 ml Almond oil.

Other Helpful Remedies

Homoeopathy

* Add about 5–10 drops of Chamomilla 3X drops to a little warmed water or milk. You could also crush a Chamomilla 6C tablet, dissolve it in 1 teaspoon of water and give this to baby from the spoon or by syringe.
* If you are breastfeeding, take the Chamomilla 6C tablet yourself; its therapeutic properties will be passed to baby via your milk. You could also express a little milk into a bottle and add Chamomilla drops to this.

Biochemic Tissue Salts

* Mag phos or Nat sulph before a feed. The tablets can be dissolved in cooled boiled water, but they also melt quickly on the tongue.

Herbal Remedies

* Simmer 1 teaspoon of dill or fennel seeds in 1 pint (600 ml) of water for 10 minutes. Strain, cool and give to baby in a bottle or on a spoon.
* Lemon Balm tisane is also soothing.
* For babies over 3 months old, mix half a teaspoon of Slippery Elm powder with a little boiled water to

make a paste. Add more water, milk or fruit juice, sweeten with a little honey if preferred and offer to baby in a bottle.
* If you are breastfeeding, have a cupful of fennel tea 3 times a day, sweetened with honey if you prefer.

Reflexology

Massage the digestive system reflex areas (*see Figure 2, page 53*).

Professional Therapies

Osteopathy

If baby regularly suffers from colic it may be a good idea to consult an osteopath. A professional treatment will possibly involve gently holding the cranium to help relieve uncomfortable strain patterns caused by the physical stress of birth or prenatal positioning. This treatment can begin about 3 weeks after birth.

Homoeopathy

Homoeopathic remedies can be very successful at treating persistent colic; all are safe for babies.

Doctor's Prescription

Over-the-counter products such as Infracol will be recommended, to be given before feeds. These help to break down any large air bubbles.

Seek help if colic persists, especially if baby screams inconsolably for hours on end or if the colicky symptoms are accompanied by persistent vomiting, diarrhoea, constipation or the absence of urine.

CONJUNCTIVITIS

Sometimes called pink eye, conjunctivitis occurs when the delicate lining covering the outer eye and eyelid becomes inflamed. This is often caused by a virus or bacterial infection, but sometimes the condition is triggered by allergies or environmental irritants such as smoke or chlorine from a swimming pool.

Typical Symptoms

Watery pink or bloodshot eyes. Discharge is clear and watery with cold viruses; bacterial infections result in a thick, yellow-green discharge; allergic conjunctivitis is accompanied by itching.

When the discharge dries during sleep the eyelids may stick together.

Practical Advice

Conjunctivitis is infectious, so take extra care when treating your baby or child's eyes. Wash your hands before and after touching them, and avoid sharing towels, bedding or clothes.

Always bathe the eyes one at a time using a clean piece of cotton wool for each eye. Wipe from the inner to the outer corner of each eye.

Naturopathy

* A sea salt solution has cleansing and mild antiseptic properties. Bathing the eyes with this simple solution keeps them free of discharge and usually clears conjunctivitis.
* Bathing baby's eyes in a little freshly expressed breastmilk can also be effective.

Herbal Remedies

* Eyebright is reputed by herbalists to be the best herb for treating the eyes. It has both cleansing and strengthening properties. Make an infusion or add a few drops of Eyebright tincture to 1 cup (240 ml) of boiled water. Allow to cool and strain. Soak a ball of cotton wool in the solution, squeeze away the excess and gently wipe the eyes. For older children you could use an eye bath.

* Chrysanthemum is the Chinese equivalent of Eyebright. Add a few drops of Chrysanthemum tincture to 1 cup (240 ml) of boiling water, or make a weak tisane by adding 1 teaspoon of dried flowers to 1 cup (240 ml) of water. Strain and use when the solution is cool.

Other Helpful Remedies

Homoeopathy

* Pulsatilla is recommended when the eyes are red, swollen and sensitive to light, with a thick yellow discharge. Give 1 tablet of the 6C potency every hour for up to 4 doses. Repeat as necessary.

* Bathe the eyes several times a day with a solution of 10 drops Euphrasia tincture in half a pint (300 ml) of cooled boiled water.

Doctor's Prescription

Antibiotic eye drops or ointment are prescribed if the conjunctivitis is due to an infection. Allergic conjunctivitis is helped by antihistamine or allergy-arresting sodium cryoglycate drops.

Seek help if conjunctivitis is still present after three days (sticky eyes usually clear up with simple bathing), if the eyes are particularly swollen and red, or if there is any loss of vision or pain in the eye.

CONSTIPATION

Constipation is often thought of as irregular or infrequent bowel movements, but with babies there are no hard-and-fast rules about how often is healthy and normal, for babies vary enormously in the number of stools they pass. Some open their bowels with every single feed, while others will happily go for more than three days without passing a stool.

Typical Symptoms

Straining and discomfort in passing stools; stools may be hard and dry.

Constipation is frequently caused by eating the wrong food, not drinking enough fluids and lack of exercise. Like adults, babies and children often suffer from constipation when they travel away from home, partly because of the change in diet but also due to the stress of moving around. Emotional upsets undoubtedly play a role in causing constipation. Your child may also become constipated if he feels rushed or hurried or simply not given enough time to go to the loo in a relaxed way. Early potty training may result in a resistance to go, which could lead to constipation.

Diet and Nutritional Therapy

* Constipation can be prevented and relieved by eating fresh fruit and vegetables. These foods are rich in natural fibre which works rather like an intestinal brush, sweeping food swiftly along the digestive tract.

* As a precautionary measure include plenty of pure fruit and vegetable purées in your baby's diet.
* Give a little prune juice to a constipated baby. Pour boiling water onto a handful of organic prunes and soak overnight, then strain and give by teaspoon or in a bottle.
* Alternatively, give baby a little strained and diluted freshly squeezed apple juice.
* If you are breastfeeding, drink at least 6 glasses of mineral water a day, and supplement with fresh fruit juice such as apple or grape. The gentle laxative effects will be passed on to baby.

Some babies become constipated when they start on solid foods. Introduce one food at a time so you know which one is causing the problem. Unripe bananas are a common cause of constipation – their skins need to have gone black before babies can digest them properly. Eggs also have a binding effect and should be avoided until baby is 12 months old.

Drinking too much milk can often lead to constipation in children. Try to replace milk with water and diluted fresh fruit juices. Rice and oat milks also make refreshing substitutes for cow's milk. Offer apples, pears, grapes, raw carrots and sticks of celery to young children to munch on as snacks between meals.

Replace white bread, biscuits, cakes and commercial cereals with wholemeal bread and pasta, brown rice and muesli-type cereals.

Try the following fresh juice blends:

* 2 large carrots and half an apple
* 1 pear and 5 oz/150 g grapes

Give no more than 5 fl oz/150 ml a day.

Other Helpful Remedies

Herbal Remedies

* Make an infusion of Liquorice or Ginger Root, sweetened with plenty of honey. Give your child sips of this 2 to 3 times a day until the constipation eases.
* For stubborn constipation you could also try giving 1 teaspoon of powdered linseeds. These could be added to cereal or soup.

Massage

Gently stroke your child's tummy in a clockwise direction. For children over 5 years old, make an aromatherapy massage oil using Marjoram, Black Pepper, Rosemary or Hyssop (singly or in combination) – 6–10 drops to 30 ml of Avocado oil.

Chinese Medicine

* Give 5–10 drops of Chinese Rhubarb root in 1 cup (240 ml) of cooled boiling water. Work two key acupressure points: Large Intestine 4 and Spleen 15 – *see Figure 1, page 13*.

Homoeopathy

* Nat mur for stools that look like 'bunny droppings'
* Nux vom for constant, ineffectual urging.

Give 1 dose of the 6C potency hourly for up to 4 doses, then 3 times a day until there is relief.

Doctor's Prescription

Different types of laxatives are used alone or in combination to retrain the intestines to work regularly.

COUGHS

Coughing is the body's natural reaction to irritation of the throat and airways. Coughs often come on after a change of weather and are particularly common during the winter months.

Coughing can be a sign of infections such as whooping cough and croup. A cough that lingers for longer than a month may progress to bronchitis, pneumonia or asthma. Babies and young children sometimes suffer from coughs when they are teething.

Typical Symptoms

A deep chesty cough often accompanies a cold and is the body's way of clearing excess mucus and phlegm in the chest and throat. A dry tickly cough is caused by inflammation in the throat and lungs, which may result from exposure to cold, dry air, extreme weather conditions or irritants in the atmosphere. Different coughs need different treatments.

Practical Advice

Being propped up with a pillow (placed under the mattress in a baby's cot) can ease a cough which is made worse by lying down.

Offer extra fluids such as water and diluted freshly squeezed juices, as they will soothe the throat and help to loosen the mucus. Do not give milk, however, as this can increase the production of mucus.

Don't let a baby become chilled, as this will aggravate a cough. Sometimes coughs are better for fresh air, but others are aggravated by cold, dry atmospheres – be watchful when you take baby outdoors.

Keep your baby or child away from smoky atmospheres.

Aromatherapy

* Lavender can help to soothe all kinds of coughs and is safe for babies under 6 months old. Gently massage the chest and back with diluted Lavender oil.

* For babies over 6 months old: Eucalyptus or Tea Tree, 3 drops essence in 30 ml of Almond oil, can also be used.

* For children over 6 years: combine any two of these essences together, for example Lavender and Eucalyptus.

* Place a few drops of your chosen essence or blend onto a tissue and tuck it into your child's pyjamas, night-dress or pillow case at night.

Homoeopathy

Try to pick the remedy that most closely matches the symptoms of your child's cough:

* Belladonna – barking cough with sore throat, often with right-sided earache or fever

* Byronia – for a dry, hacking cough which comes on slowly and in fits. Accompanied by feeling 'fluey' and extremely irritable. Better for lying down or sitting still, worse for moving around.

* Hepar sulph – for a loose choking or suffocating cough which can become croupy. Accompanied by feeling chilly and sweaty, disliking any draughts. Worse for breathing in cold air, being uncovered or getting cold. Thirsty for hot drinks.

* Phosphorus – for a dry, hacking, tickling cough that leaves the sufferer hoarse. Burning pains and a feeling of pressure and tightness in the chest when

coughing. Nose can be running or blocked up. Worse in the mornings and evenings.

* Pulsatilla – loose in the morning and dry at night; with green nasal discharge and left-sided earache.

Give 1 dose of the 30C potency, wait to see if there is any improvement and, if so, follow up with 1 dose a day for the next 2 days.

For long-standing, persistent or recurrent coughs it is advisable to consult a professional homoeopath.

Other Helpful Remedies

Diet and Nutritional Therapy

* Freshly squeezed lemon juice and honey in hot water makes a soothing cough remedy.
* You could also try the following fresh juice blend: 4 tangerines, half a lemon and 1 teaspoon of honey. Give 5 fl oz/150 ml a day.
* Cabbage and Brussels sprouts are reputedly good for preventing and easing coughs.

Herbal Remedies

* Use plenty of garlic and thyme in your cooking.
* Give Little Ones' Cough Syrup (*see page 31*): 1 teaspoon 3 times a day.
* Alternatively, try Elderflower Syrup (*see page 31*).

Chinese Medicine

In Chinese medicine coughs are usually associated with an excess of *yin* which needs to be calmed. A simple home remedy for a dry cough is warm milk and honey. For a cough with excessive mucus try a warming ginger tea (1 teaspoon grated ginger steeped in boiling water, strained and sweetened with honey).

To ease a coughing fit apply pressure to the Kidney 27 acupressure point – *see Figure 1, page 13*.

Biochemic Tissue Salts

* Combination J: 2 tablets every hour until the cough eases, then 3 times daily.
* Some babies need careful nursing through bad coughs and may need special medical attention if self-help measures do not bring relief within 48 hours.

Doctor's Prescription

Unexplained coughing that is not the result of an obvious chest infection may be due to asthma. Typically childhood asthma can present with coughing at night, during exercise or in response to irritants such as cigarette smoke.

Seek help if your baby cannot keep fluids or solids down because of coughing, if the cough is accompanied by difficulty breathing, wheezing or chest pain, or if baby has a bluish tinge around the face, mouth and tongue or becomes abnormally drowsy.

CRADLE CAP

Cradle cap varies from being flaky white patches mainly on the top of the scalp to a thick, yellowish scaling covering the whole scalp. It is caused by the over-activity of the sebaceous (oil-producing) glands which lie at the root of hair follicles.

Most babies seem to go through a period of getting cradle cap, usually when they begin to grow hair. It can be made worse by using a harsh shampoo and not rinsing properly. It is easy to treat with natural remedies.

Aromatherapy

* Make up one of the scalp oils listed below; massage a little into baby's scalp when it is dry. Left on overnight it will soften the cradle cap, you can then rub the scales off when washing baby's hair next morning. Resist the temptation to pick the scales off with your fingertips.
* Under 6 months: plain vegetable oil
* For babies over 6 months: 3–4 drops Lemon or Eucalyptus essence in 30 ml Almond or Avocado oil
* For babies over 12 months: 3 drops Lemon Eucalyptus and 3 drops Geranium in 30 ml Almond or Avocado oil.

Diet and Nutritional Therapy

* Cradle cap has been linked to low levels of vitamin B_6. Levels of this vitamin are often low during pregnancy, and if supplies also dwindle after birth baby may not get all the vitamin B_6 he needs.
* If breastfeeding, enrich your diet with foods that supply plentiful amounts of this vitamin. These include fish, whole grain cereals, bananas, avocados, nuts, seeds and some leafy vegetables.
* The mineral zinc is also important to the formation of healthy skin; lack of it may be a contributing factor in cradle cap. Zinc requirements increase in pregnancy and lactation, but are not always fulfilled. Zinc-rich foods are lamb, chicken, ginger root, eggs, shrimp, potatoes, carrots, beans, parsley and most nuts, especially pecans, peanuts, almonds, walnuts and hazelnuts.

Herbal Remedy

* After washing with a natural soap shampoo, rinse the scalp with an infusion of Burdock Root.

CROUP

An acute infection of the larynx (voice box) which commonly affects children under the age of 5. Croup can be the aftermath of a cold and cough, or may be due to an infection or allergy to something in the environment, possibly dust, house dust mites or mould spores. This condition can also be stress-related.

Typical Symptoms

Similar to those of a cough and cold, with a runny nose and slight fever. A baby or child may sound hoarse, have a harsh, barking cough and may experience breathing difficulties.

Hydrotherapy

Steam treatment is the traditional and most effective way to relieve bouts of coughing. Make your child's bedroom as humid as possibly by placing bowls of steaming water near radiators (providing they are completely out of your child's reach), boil a kettle in the room or use a humidifier.

The bathroom is a good place to go if baby has a bad attack of coughing because you can fill the room with steam very quickly by running hot water from the shower or bath taps. Sit and cuddle your child until the cough eases.

Mustard footbaths can also be beneficial. Dissolve 1 teaspoon of mustard powder in a basin of warm water and encourage your child to soak his feet in the bath for 5 to 10 minutes.

Homoeopathy

* Aconite is the first choice. Give the 30C potency if your child is breathless and panicky, 1 dose immediately and another 30 minutes later.

* If Aconite brings no relief and the child develops a loud, very dry, barking cough which sounds like sawing wood, and he loses his voice, try Spongia if the attacks occur before midnight and Hepar Sulph if they come during the early hours of the morning. Give 1 or 2 doses of the 30C potency as required.

For recurrent bouts of croup it is a good idea to consult a professional homoeopath.

Other Helpful Remedies

Herbal Remedy

* Try giving teaspoons of soothing Chamomile, Peppermint or Catnip tea with 5 to 10 drops of Lobelia tincture, sweetened with honey if your child will take it.

Diet and Nutritional Therapy

* Give sips of freshly squeezed lemon juice diluted with hot water and sweetened with honey.

Doctor's Prescription

Severely distressed children may need to be admitted to hospital. Babies in such distress will use their chest wall and abdominal (tummy) muscles to aid breathing. If you see your baby or child doing this, consult your doctor.

Seek help if symptoms are not eased by the steam treatment and your baby or child's breathing is laboured. Emergency care may be needed which involves administering oxygen in a special chamber.

CRYING (IN BABIES)

Crying is a baby's first language and, as you get to know your baby, you will begin to distinguish between different cries and understand what they mean.

Babies cry when they are wet, cold or hungry, if they have wind or an upset tummy, if they are bored or lonely or if they are threatening for an illness. Piercing and persistent cries usually mean a baby is in pain or distressed. Feeble, whingy crying often means baby is miserable or feeling slightly unwell.

It is also normal for breastfed babies to cry quite a lot early on; this should cease once a feeding routine has been established.

In general, happy babies do not cry a lot whereas those who are anxious, need some care and attention or are ill tend to be more tearful. There are also times when babies cry for no apparent reason; theories abound as to why this should be.

Some say our Western style of baby care may be partly to blame. Babies instinctively wish to be held; being placed in a cot in another room deprives them of this closeness. Crying is the only way they can tell us what they want; simply picking them up often works a treat.

In most native cultures babies are constantly carried around, tied onto their mother's back or hip with a shawl. Babies often sleep with their parents or are taken into bed to feed until they are about a year old, too.

A baby's tears may also signal a mental growth spurt. Neurological studies show there are dramatic changes in a child's brain during the first 18 months. While these changes mean baby is able to learn many new skills, the process is nevertheless bewildering and baby's natural reaction is to seek comfort and security in a parent's arms.

Dr Hetty Van de Rijt and Professor Frans Plooij, child development specialists at the Universities of Amsterdam and Groningen, have identified seven mental growth spurts in the first 12 months of life and say they can predict when fretful times are likely. These are at around 5, 8, 12, 15, 23, 34 and 42 weeks of age. Each clingy, crying period can last several days, sometimes several weeks, with a particularly stormy week in the middle. After each developmental leap baby should settle down and try out his new skills. (For more information, please consult the References and Further Reading chapter.)

Practical Advice

Try all the obvious things like feeding, changing baby's nappy, cuddling, adding or taking away clothes.

Babies can get frustrated and tearful when they are bored; try going for a walk or giving your baby some interesting things to look at or play with.

Homoeopathy

Homoeopathic remedies can help those situations where anxiety and tearfulness escalate into excessive crying or clinging. Choose the remedy that best suits your baby's particular disposition.

* Borax – for nervous babies who are easily startled by sudden noises and who are tearful at night. They may wake screaming from the slightest noise or for no apparent reason, as if from a nightmare. They hate downward motion and scream on being rocked or put down in their cots. If asleep when you place them in their cots they wake immediately. They do not like being jigged up and down in the air. They are particularly

irritable before passing a stool, reverting dramatically to cheerfulness straight afterwards. Children who need Borax will be jumpy and anxious at night.

* Chamomilla – for irritable, angry babies, especially when teething. They are tearful, often screaming with pain. They insist on being carried and cry loudly when held still or put down. Toddlers who need Chamomilla will whine, scream and refuse to be comforted. They become spiteful and may hit parents. They ask for things which they then throw across the room. Worse from 9 p.m. to midnight.

* Lycopodium – these babies may sleep well at night but cry all day. They are irritable in the mornings after a sleep. They are often fearful of strangers. As toddlers they can be irritable and dictatorial, having tantrums if contradicted. They are generally difficult to live with.

* Pulsatilla – clingy and dependent, particularly when sick when they also become irritable and whiny. Many babies go through a Pulsatilla stage when they are weepy and want to be carried around all the time.

Give 1 dose of the 30C potency; if this brings some relief repeat for up to 3 doses.

If baby does not respond to the remedy you choose, it may be a good idea to consult a professional who can select the most suitable constitutional remedy.

Other Helpful Remedies

Herbal Remedy

* Chamomile is a soothing remedy for crying babies. Add a drop or two to baby's bath and use in a vaporizer to fragrance baby's bedroom.

Flower Remedies

* Pear blossom (Master's Flower Essences) – for crying related to birth complications, shock and all forms of emotional or physical crisis
* Rescue Remedy (Bach Flower Remedies) or Five Flowers Remedy (Healing Herbs) – a good all-purpose remedy for crying that results from any kind of upset or trauma
* White Hyacinth (Petite Fleur Essences) – for feelings of uncertainty and insecurity relating to the shock and trauma of childbirth.

Professional Therapy

Diet and Nutritional Therapy

Dietary factors may be responsible if babies cry a good deal, are irritable, miserable, tearful, difficult to soothe with cuddles and wake frequently during the night, especially if they suffer from bad nappy rash, bowel disturbances and frequent infections.

* Babies can be allergic to cow's milk and often fare better when given a substitute such as goat's milk or soya milk.
* Low zinc levels have been found in babies who are irritable, tearful, mentally lethargic and difficult to soothe. Research has shown that babies waking one or more times a night between midnight and 7 a.m. improve their sleep pattern when given 12 mg of elemental zinc. Breastmilk is a particularly good source of zinc.

If you have tried everything and suspect your baby's crying may be diet-related do consult a qualified nutritionist for more specific advice.

Osteopathy

Treatment focusing on the cranium often works wonders.

Doctor's Prescription

A full physical examination may be reassuring and helps to exclude any medical cause.

Seek help if your baby's cries are persistent and he seems to be in pain.

See also **Anxiety**

CUTS AND SCRATCHES

Cuts and scratches are an inevitable part of childhood; most minor ones heal quickly on their own provided proper care is taken to prevent them becoming infected.

Always clean any wound thoroughly, washing the broken skin with warm soap and water to remove any dirt.

Aromatherapy

* Essential oils make excellent antiseptics. Add 2 drops Lavender to a basin of warm water (for babies over 6 months old you could also add 1 drop Tea Tree, a particularly powerful antiseptic). Soak cotton wool in this solution and dab onto the wound.
* If the cut is still bleeding put a drop of neat Lavender onto a plaster and cover it up. When the bleeding subsides, expose to the fresh air for as long as possible, even if this just means taking the plaster off at night.
* For deep cuts repeat the bathing several times a day until the wound starts to heal.

Herbal Remedies

* You can make your own Calendula oil for rubbing into cuts and scratches. Fill a jam jar with marigold flowers. Cover with olive oil and leave to steep in the sunlight for a day (alternatively, warm gently in an airing cupboard overnight). Strain before use.
* Use the Cream for Drawing Out Glass, Thorns and Splinters (*see page 31*).

Homoeopathy

* Calendula is the number one first-aid remedy for healing cuts and wounds. Taken internally it stimulates the formation of healthy scar tissue (without lumps). Give 1 dose of the 30C potency immediately and once a day for the next 2 days.
* Bathe cuts in a solution made from 1 teaspoon of Calendula tincture added to 1 cup (240 ml) of cooled boiled water.
* Calendula ointment smoothed into a cut soothes and speeds skin healing.
* Hypercal ointment can be helpful if the cut is causing a lot of pain.

Doctor's Prescription

Most cuts and scratches heal by themselves. Dirty wounds should be cleaned and dressed by a nurse. Children should be vaccinated against tetanus, as contaminated soil may contain tetanus spores.

CYSTITIS

This condition is due to an inflammation of the urinary system most often caused by a bacterial infection. Antibiotics, stress and a poor diet can also cause cystitis.

Typical Symptoms

Frequent urination accompanied by a burning or stinging sensation. There is often an overwhelming urge to go again straight after passing urine. Urine may have a strong odour or appear dark and cloudy. There may be pain in the abdominal area.

Boys and girls can get cystitis, but it is more common in girls because of their anatomy: the urethra, which leads to the bladder, shares virtually the same opening as the vagina and is very close to the anus. Many infections in the urinary tract area are caused by intestinal germs such as *E. coli*. Taking special care to wipe from front to back is a good preventative measure.

Practical Advice

Discourage your child from holding on when he needs to spend a penny.

Avoid using scented bubble baths, soaps and baby wipes, as the chemicals in them can be irritant. Choose plain (unscented, uncoloured) toilet paper for the same reason.

Diet and Nutritional Therapy

* Encourage your child to drink lots of mineral water, at least 8 glasses a day, to flush the infection from the bladder.
* Cranberries are renowned for helping to prevent and

relieve cystitis. They produce hippuric acid in the urine, which acidifies the urinary tract and inhibits the growth of bacteria. Give sugar-free cranberry juice to drink twice a day, or serve the freshly cooked fruit. If these are rejected you can buy cranberry tablets from most healthfood stores.

* Lemon barley water can be soothing. The best kind is home-made: Boil a little barley with some slices of lemon, strain and sweeten with honey and put in the fridge to chill.

* Helpful foods to include in your child's diet are avocado and raspberries as they reduce a proliferation of bacteria in the bladder. Celery and parsley are naturally diuretic. Garlic and onions are antibiotic, so mix them with other vegetables, sprinkle with olive oil and bake in the oven.

* Try the following fresh juice blend: 1 apple, 1 pear and 3 fl oz/90 ml of water. Give 5 fl oz/150 ml a day.

* A traditional Chinese remedy for cystitis is watermelon juice – give large slices of watermelon to suck.

* During an attack of cystitis try to eliminate sugar, refined carbohydrates, dried fruits and yeast-containing foods (bread, croissants, Marmite, vinegar and pickles) from the diet.

* A broad-spectrum multi-vitamin and mineral supplement providing beta carotene, vitamin E, B complex vitamins, vitamin C and bioflavonoids, calcium, zinc and magnesium can help to clear and prevent recurrent attacks of cystitis.

* If your child is given antibiotics for the infection it is important to restore the healthy bacteria destroyed by

the drugs. Give at least one carton of live, unsweetened yoghurt (containing *Lactobacillus acidophilus*) a day for the next few weeks.

Homoeopathy

* Berberis – for burning pain even when not urinating
* Cantharis – when the desire to urinate is urgent, frequent and ineffectual. Burning pains before and after come on suddenly and are violent and spasmodic. Worse for cold drinks despite having a great thirst.
* Sarsaparilla – may pass urine without feeling pain, until the end when pains are cutting. Slow and feeble urination
* Staphisagria – burning pain continues after urination.

Give 1 dose of the 6C potency every 30 minutes for up to 5 doses. Repeat as necessary.

Seek professional homoeopathic treatment if cystitis is recurrent.

Other Helpful Remedies

Aromatherapy

Massage the lower back and tummy with a salve containing Sandalwood essential oil.

Hydrotherapy

Give your child coolish baths with seasalt added. Apply cold compresses to the lower abdomen.

Herbal Remedy

* Children's urinary problems often respond well to a combination of Cornsilk and Marshmallow Root. Prepare by simmering $1/2$ oz/15 g of Marshmallow Root in 1 pint (600 ml) of boiling water for 15 minutes. Make an infusion of Cornsilk by steeping 2 teaspoons in 1 cup (240 ml) of boiling water for 5 minutes. Combine the two infusions, sweeten with honey and give as sips throughout the day.

Doctor's Prescription

Cystitis in children under 3 years old always needs to be investigated to ensure that the kidneys are not involved.

Investigations involve scans of the kidneys and renal tract. If treatment is necessary antibiotics are given in small doses long term (until 3 or 4 years of age) to protect the kidneys.

Occasionally an operation is necessary to correct an anatomical defect in the ureter (collecting duct into the bladder).

Seek help if there is feverishness and any pain in the kidney area. It is wise to consult your doctor in order that a sample of urine can be analysed to pinpoint the offending bacteria. Occasionally cystitis in children can be caused by micro-organisms such as chlamydia which need specialist treatment.

D

DEPRESSION

Children can feel depressed from time to time, just like adults. It is quite normal for any of us to go through periods of feeling miserable providing it is only for a short while and there is a tangible reason. Your child may be disappointed by exam results or by the thought of going back to school after the summer holidays.

Sometimes depression is caused by pent-up anger or the inability to cry. Feelings of isolation and loneliness may also bring on depression. In some instances, depression can arise when our physical vitality is low after an illness or as a result of poor nutrition. Natural remedies can help to lift the spirits and improve mood, but the best way to deal with your child's depression is to pay special attention to him. Try to find out what is causing the problem, discuss it and attempt to provide a solution.

Herbal Remedies

* St John's Wort (*Hypericum perforatum*), sometimes referred to as the sunshine herb, may help to lift the spirits. Research conducted in Germany and reported in the *British Medical Journal* suggests that St John's Wort can be as effective as orthodox anti-depressants in treating mild to moderate depression, without the adverse side-effects of drugs.

* Add drops of Hypericum tincture to fruit juice or mineral water, or give herbal tablets (1 tablet 3 times a day).

* Children's Stress Formula (*see page 32*): 10 drops in 6 fl oz/180 ml cooled boiled water 2 times a day (morning and evening).

Flower Remedies

* Gorse (Bach Flower Remedies, Healing Herbs) – for times when life seems a misery, bringing hopelessness and despair. For those who feel resigned to feeling that nothing can be done to help.

* Larch (Bach Flower Remedies, Healing Herbs) – for those who are full of self-doubt and who lack self-confidence, leading to feelings of depression and despondency.

* Mustard (Bach Flower Remedies, Healing Herbs) – for overwhelming black clouds of depression of unknown origin, causing deep sadness and melancholy that lifts as suddenly as it descends.

* Red Rose (Petite Fleur) – for gloominess and occasional depression. Replaces these feelings with enthusiasm and joy.

* Valerian (Findhorn Flower Essences) – lifts the spirits and rekindles delight and happiness in living. Restores a sense of humour and fun.

Give 2 drops of essence 3 times daily until the depression lifts.

Other Helpful Remedies
Aromatherapy

* Sweet Orange or Mandarin can lighten the hearts of young children. Use it in the bath, in a massage oil, with a few drops on a pillow case and as a vapour around the house. For children over 7 years old you can use Rose and Sandalwood too, perhaps making a blend using 4 drops of each to 30 ml of almond oil.
* For speedy benefits massage the aromatherapy oil into the feet and hands, concentrating your attention on the endocrine system reflex points.

Professional Therapy
Homoeopathy

A qualified homoeopath can often help to relieve depression.

Doctor's Prescription

Anti-depressant drugs are not commonly prescribed for children.
Treatment more often centres around behavioural and family therapy with a child psychologist or psychiatrist.

Seek help if you suspect your child may be suffering from chronic depression. Tell-tale signs are lethargy, being withdrawn and uncommunicative, difficulty sleeping and then getting up in the morning, an inability to concentrate and loss of interest in life.

DIARRHOEA

Diarrhoea is usually a sign that the body is trying to get rid of a bacterium, virus or irritant substance. Food poisoning is one of the commonest causes of diarrhoea. It can also be due to a change of diet, anxiety, or treatment with antibiotics. Persistent diarrhoea may be the result of a food allergy or intolerance and will need specialist treatment (*see* **Food Allergies**).

Small babies with diarrhoea need to be watched carefully as they can quickly become dehydrated. If diarrhoea persists for more than two days, do consult your doctor.

Typical Symptoms

Frequent passing of loose, watery stools which often smell unpleasant and are pale in colour. Ranges from a mild bout lasting a few hours to a violent and prolonged attack accompanied by stomach cramps, nausea or vomiting which leaves the sufferer feeling weak, shivery and aching.

Prevention

Be scrupulous about cleanliness when preparing food. Always wash fruits and vegetables thoroughly and rinse in filtered water. Make sure poultry and meats are well cooked. Frozen chickens need to be completely thawed before they are put in the oven to reduce the risk of salmonella food poisoning. Never give your child uncooked (or even only slightly uncooked) eggs.

When travelling abroad it is best to avoid certain foods. Salads are particularly risky as they can become contaminated with *E. coliform* bacteria, the bug most responsible for diarrhoea. Fruits are fine if washed and peeled, but do not buy those displayed on the street as they are often contaminated by flies and other people's touching them.

Soak fruit in sterilized water (i.e. water treated with Milton tablets).

Avoid the local milk and any ice-cream or yoghurt made from it. In many countries milk is unpasteurized and, even in those where it is, standards are not always that high.

Use bottled mineral water instead of tap water and make sure the seal is intact. Avoid ice in drinks as it is usually made from tap water.

Before travelling give your child lots of 'live' natural yoghurt to ensure that there are plenty of healthy bacteria in the intestines. You could add a $1/2$ teaspoon of powdered *Lactobacillus acidophilus* (available from healthfood stores) to an evening milky drink for two to three weeks prior to going on holiday.

Treatment

Do not give solids to eat during an attack of diarrhoea, especially if accompanied by vomiting.

To prevent dehydration it is vital to replace lost fluids. Make sure your baby or child takes small sips of cooled boiled water at frequent intervals throughout the day.

If diarrhoea lasts longer than 24 hours make a special drink to replenish lost salts: Add 1 teaspoon of salt and 2 dessertspoons of sugar to 2 pints (1.2 litres) of boiled water; add 1 pint (600 ml) of orange or lemon juice. Give your child a glass of this mixture every hour until symptoms subside.

After a dose of diarrhoea give small, simple meals several times a day. Apples and carrots help to soothe the digestive system. They are best served raw and grated, steamed or stewed.

The freshly squeezed juice of 1 apple diluted with 4 fl oz/120 ml is ideal for small babies.

Other good foods are well-ripened bananas and simple vegetable soups. Plain 'live' natural yoghurt sweetened with honey will help to replenish healthy intestinal bacteria.

Boost the body's healthy bacteria by giving a supplement such as bifidophilus which contains both acidophilus and bifidus bacteria. Give 1 capsule a day for a month after a bout of diarrhoea.

Other Helpful Remedies
Herbal Remedies

* Herbalists recommend Raspberry leaves for diarrhoea and stomach upsets in small children. Add 1 teaspoon to 1 cup (240 ml) of boiling water, steep for 5 minutes and strain. Sweeten with honey to taste and give as sips.
* Herbalists may also recommend giving frequent sips of Meadowseet infusion or tincture, diluted in water.
* Slippery Elm is very soothing and settling. Mix $1/2$ – 1 teaspoon with a little boiled water to make a paste. Dilute with a little more water until it is fluid enough to drink. Sweeten with a bit of honey if preferred.

Chinese Medicine

Diarrhoea in babies is seen as a sign of imbalance in the spleen and stomach meridians. Chinese dandelion is a traditional herbal remedy for treating this kind of diarrhoea.

Add at least 5 drops of tincture to 1 cup (240 ml) of boiling water, leave to cool and give as sips. To enhance the benefits you could also rub Cinnamon or Ginger oil into the stomach area.

Work the Spleen 15 acupressure point – *see Figure 1, page 13*.

Aromatherapy

Several essential oils can help to relieve diarrhoea when massaged into the tummy:

* For babies under 6 months old: 1–2 drops of Lavender essential oil in 30 ml of Almond oil.
* For babies over 1 year old: blend Lavender, Eucalyptus, Geranium and Peppermint (1 drop of each in 30 ml of Almond oil).
* For children over 5 years old: add Sandalwood to the blend. This time use 2 drops of each essence in 30 ml of Almond oil.

Homoeopathy

Arsenicum album is the number one remedy for food poisoning. The symptom profile is profuse diarrhoea accompanied by a burning and colicky stomach, restlessness, anxiety and chilliness. Give 1 dose of the 6C potency every 30 minutes for up to 4 doses; repeat if necessary.

Reflexology

Work the digestive system reflex areas on the feet and hands (*see Figure 2, page 53*).

Doctor's Prescription

If diarrhoea persists for more than a few days, your doctor may request a stool sample for analysis to detect the particular bacteria responsible and then prescribe according to the findings.

Seek help if diarrhoea persists and fluids are not kept down; if your baby or child looks very pale and seems exhausted; if your child complains of acute abdominal pain which does not respond to the above treatments and is getting steadily worse. It could be a sign of a more serious condition such as appendicitis.

E

EARACHE AND EAR INFECTIONS

Earache is frequently caused by a bacterial or viral infection resulting from a cold or sore throat. The build-up of catarrh in the middle ear presses against the eardrum causing considerable pain. Ear infections can also result from poking things (such as a pencil or cotton bud) into the ear, a build-up of ear wax and, perhaps more unexpectedly, from blowing extra hard through both nostrils.

If your baby seems to have earache, avoid the temptation to clean his ears and don't take him out into a cold wind.

If your child is feverish and very miserable ask your doctor to check his ears for infection. Left unchecked, an infection can perforate the eardrum and possibly cause permanent damage.

Typical Symptoms

Throbbing or stabbing pain in the ears that is often worse for lying down. Earache can occur during a cold characterized by a runny nose, slight fever and sore throat. Babies may rub their heads, pull at their ears and cry inconsolably, especially in the evenings. They may also suffer from sickness and diarrhoea. Young children with earache tend to be tearful, clingy, whingy and miserable.

Diet and Nutritional Therapy

Breastfeeding is a good preventative measure. Research shows that children who are breastfed experience fewer ear infections than those who are not.

* Naturopaths believe that cow's milk encourages the production of catarrh; their approach shows that recurrent earaches can sometimes be relieved by substituting this with goat's, sheep's or soya milk.
* Encourage your child to drink plenty of fluids.

Aromatherapy

* An old-fashioned remedy for earache involves putting a piece of cotton wool soaked in slightly warm (not hot) extra-virgin olive oil into the ear. To enhance the beneficial effect of this remedy, add 1 drop of Lavender and 1 drop of Chamomile essence to 1 teaspoon of olive oil, mix well and soak the cotton wool in this mixture. Make sure the cotton wool ball is big enough so that it cannot be pushed right into the ear.
* For children over 7 years old: add 1 drop of Basil essence to this blend.

Other Helpful Remedies

Naturopathy

For immediate relief try holding a warm hot water bottle wrapped in a towel to the ear.

Herbal Remedies

* Mullein and Yarrow are traditional herbal remedies for earache. Mullein flowers steeped in oil have antibacterial and pain-relieving properties. Massage with this oil around the outer ear, particularly behind the ears. A few drops can also be placed into the ear.
* St John's Wort oil is another beneficial remedy.
* An infusion of Yarrow can be applied on cotton wool as a hot compress to the outside of the ear.

Homoeopathy

* Pulsatilla is the number one remedy for childhood ear infections where discharges from the ear are thick, bland and yellow-green and the left ear is mainly affected. The ear complaint may come on after the sufferer has got his feet wet or chilled. The symptoms and the patients themselves will be very changeable. Your child will be moody, tearful and crave company, clingy and whingy. He will have no thirst and feel worse for being in a stuffy room. Mood improves in the fresh air. Better for bathing, crying, movement. Worse for twilight, wet and windy weather.
* Belladonna – for throbbing pains where the external ear is red and hot, children become wide-eyed and delirious. Right ear is usually affected.
* Chamomilla – the sufferer will be inconsolable and

furious from the pain, cannot be soothed, pain worse for cold air and draughts.

Give the 6C potency every 15 minutes for up to 4 doses.

Chinese Medicine

Place 1–2 drops of diluted Peppermint oil into the ear. Work the Small Intestine 19 acupressure point – *see Figure 1, page 13*.

Professional Therapy

Osteopathy

Recurrent earaches can sometimes be resolved by cranial osteopathy, particularly if they began after an injury or bump to the head or spine, which can affect the drainage of the ears.

Doctor's Prescription

Paracetamol is usually recommended to relieve the pain and reduce the fever. Antibiotics may be prescribed to clear an infection.

ECZEMA

Infantile atopic eczema is most common in young babies where there is a history of asthma or hay fever in the family. It affects around 15 per cent of babies and young children. Many appear to grow out of this condition as they get older.

Eczema can be triggered and exacerbated by a wide range of irritants. These include dust, house dust mites, pet hairs and feathers, food allergies, chemicals in swimming pools, wool, synthetic fibres, biological washing powders, perfumed soaps and bubble baths. Flare-ups often occur during times of stress, as a result of a fever associated with a viral illness, and during teething in babies.

This is a chronic condition which needs to be treated both internally and externally.

Typical Symptoms

Inflammation of the skin accompanied by itchiness, redness and sometimes small blisters, scales or scabs. Often seen as red, scaly patches on the cheeks, behind the ears and in skin folds such as the elbows, knees, armpits and wrists.

Ranges from a mild condition characterized by a few dry itchy patches to a severe form affecting the whole body. Eczema may be dry or weepy. It can also become infected, which causes the condition to spread.

Diet and Nutritional Therapy

* The omega 3 and 6 series essential fatty acids have been found to be particularly helpful in treating eczema. Omega 3 fatty acids are supplied by oily fish such as mackerel, sardines, herrings and salmon. Evening Primrose oil and Star flower oils are some of the richest known sources of the Omega 6 fatty acids.

* Try giving 2 to 4 500-mg capsules of Evening Primrose oil and 2 capsules of Cod liver oil a day. The vitamin A in cod liver oil may also be helpful, as this nutrient plays a role in keeping skin soft and healthy. The contents of these capsules can be tipped into a nightly bottle of milk for babies.

* Many eczema sufferers cannot tolerate cow's milk. Good substitutes are goat's and sheep's milk, soya milk, almond milk *(see recipe on page 159)* and rice milk for children over 2 years old.

* Other possible allergens implicated in eczema are wheat, corn, oranges and all preservatives, colourants and additives. It is important that you consult a professional nutritionist before excluding more than one or two foods from your child's diet.

* Eczema sufferers often have low levels of certain nutrients, in particular zinc, a mineral needed for the formation of healthy tissue, calcium and vitamin B_6. A broad spectrum vitamin and mineral supplement may be helpful.

Chinese Medicine

Medical trials carried out at the Great Ormond Street Hospital in London have shown Chinese herbs to be very beneficial in treating eczema. Some typical herbs used are Oriental wormwood, Chinese gentian and peony root. Chinese herbalists recommend personal prescriptions tailored towards each individual and taken under supervision.

Tincture of nettle is a safe home remedy to try. Add 5 drops or more to 1 cup (240 ml) of boiling water, leave to cool and give as sips. Externally, marigold or chrysanthemum flowers can be made into an infusion and added to the bath or applied as a compress to the affected areas.

Other Helpful Remedies

Homoeopathy

Eczema should be treated with a professionally prescribed constitutional remedy. However, the following homoeopathic remedies may bring temporary relief:

* Graphites – for cracked skin with a yellow oozing discharge

* Rhus tox – for burning, itching and stinging rashes; worse for cold, after scratching.
* Sulphur – for burning red, hot and itchy skin.

Give 1 dose of the 6C potency morning and evening.

Every morning and evening apply Calendula cream to dry, rough patches. Hypericum cream is recommended if the skin is scratched and bleeding.

Aromatherapy

* Make a therapeutic bath by tossing a handful of sea salt in with the running water and adding a few drops of Lavender (*see recommendations, page 6*).
* For children over 7 years: a blend of Lavender and Bergamot.
* After bathing massage skin with a diluted blend of Chamomile, Lavender and Geranium in a base of Rosehip oil.

Hydrotherapy

Add 5 tablespoons of oatmeal to a cheesecloth or muslin bag and soak in the bath water. This helps to relieve itching and soothe the skin.

Relaxation

Like asthma, eczema is a stress-related condition. Eczema can be triggered and exacerbated by emotional upsets. Try to identify the sources of stress in your child's life and make sure he has plenty of time for relaxing pursuits such as reading books and playing games. You could also try guided visualization.

Flower Remedies

* Billy Goat Plum (Australian Bush Flower Essences) – for stress-related skin conditions.
* Vanilla Leaf (Pacific Essences) – for skin disorders relating to lack of self-esteem.

Herbal Remedy

* Immune Balancing Formula (*see page 32*) will help to calm an overactive immune system.

Doctor's Prescription

Flare-ups are minimized by the use of emollients for the bath such as Balneum, and moisturizers such as Aqueous cream on a daily basis. Both can be prescribed by your doctor. Steroid creams are given for flare-ups but should only be used for a short time, as long-term they can cause skin damage.

See also **Allergies**

F

FEEDING PROBLEMS

Children's erratic eating habits are usually more distressing for their parents! We have fixed ideas about how much children should eat, and tend to be overly concerned with average growth rates and weights. Left to their own instincts children will eat what their bodies need, providing, of course, they are offered a good variety of nutritious home-made foods.

Children's appetites often vary from day to day and from week to week. There are times when they always seem to be hungry, and others when they not that interested in food. In most children, periods of heavy eating usually coincide with growth spurts.

Appetite may also be a good indicator of general health. It is normal for babies and children to go off their food when they are sickening for something or feeling unwell.

The worst thing you can do is push your child into eating

when he is not hungry. Avoid the temptation to buy speciality foods in an attempt to seduce your child into eating. It will only create a desire for foods which have no real place in a wholesome diet. If your child repeatedly refuses a certain food, it may not agree with him, in which case it is best to offer alternatives.

Foods such as milk, cheese and red meat may be rich in certain nutrients but they are not essential for good health; there are many other foods which supply the same nutrients in equally plentiful amounts.

Never try to bribe your child into eating, or use food as a reward. Eating is about nourishment and pleasure. To use it for any other purpose may sow the seeds for emotional problems with food in the future.

Even if you are worried about how much and what your child is eating, try to conceal it. Once aware of your concern, a child is likely to play on it for the sake of getting what he wants.

Diet and Nutritional Therapy

* Loss of appetite may be a symptom of nutritional deficiencies. In children a lack of iron is linked to poor appetite and growth as well as a reduced resistance to infection.

* When zinc levels are low the senses of taste and smell are dulled so that foods taste bland and eating becomes unenjoyable. Low levels of this mineral are also associated with slow growth.

* To encourage a healthy appetite it is better that your child eats small quantities of a variety of different nutrient-rich foods than larger amounts of 'junk food'. It may be helpful to give a broad spectrum vitamin and mineral supplement daily if your child is a poor eater, lacks vitality or is recovering from an illness.

Biochemic Tissue Salts

* Calc phos helps in the assimilation of nutrients and is recommended for low vitality and digestive problems.

Herbal Remedy

* Happy Child Formula (*see page 33*) may be helpful: 10 drops in 6 fl oz/180 ml water 3 times a day until the appetite improves.

If you are genuinely concerned about your child's growth levels, a food allergy or nutritional deficiency, it is important to consult a qualified nutritionist.

FEVER AND HIGH TEMPERATURE

A fever is defined as a body temperature over 98.6°F (37°C) measured by mouth. A temperature rise is usually a sign that the body is fighting an infection, such as a cold, flu, ear infection or sore throat. It may also result from over-exposure to heat or cold and, in children, in response to a shock or emotional disturbance.

Typical Symptoms

High temperature characterized by feeling hot and flushed, sometimes with shivering, thirst and weakness. Just before a fever your child may whine, become clingy and regress to baby-like behaviour or become quiet and withdrawn. Occasionally a child with a fever may throw a tantrum or become delirious. While distressing, this is not dangerous.

Although a normal temperature is said to be 98.6°F (37°C) body temperatures normally vary up to one full degree over the course of a day, ranging from 97.5°F (36.2°C) to 99.5°F (37.5°C) with lower readings in the morning and higher ones in the afternoon.

Temperature is normally controlled by a 'thermostat' in a part of the brain called the hypothalamus. When a child has an infection, the white blood cells fighting the infection send chemical messages (interleukins) to the hypothalamus. The thermostat is then raised to help the white blood cells do their job. Fevers kill many germs including strep pneumonia, the bacteria responsible for ear infections.

For each 1°c rise in temperature the healing reactions of the body are speeded up by approximately 10 per cent. The heart beats faster (carrying blood around the body more quickly), breathing quickens (increasing oxygen uptake) and perspiration increases (helping the body to cool down).

Natural therapists regard a fever as a good sign, as it shows the body is fighting an illness. It is quite normal for healthy infants and children to run a temperature of 103°c (39.5°c) during an infection for several days without any dangers. Children generally run higher temperatures than adults.

A high temperature may also result from over-bundling your baby. Babies can't shake off their blankets or remove their clothes so they get over-heated just from being overdressed in a hot environment. If your baby feels hot to the touch it is a good idea to try taking off some layers to see if his temperature drops before assuming he is ill.

Teething babies may run a slight temperature but it is normally no greater than 101°F (38.4°c)

Taking Your Child's Temperature

Place a thermometer under your child's tongue or tuck it under his armpit for 5 minutes. Electronic varieties are safer than the old-fashioned mercury thermometers, which your child might accidentally bite. A fever strip only gives a rough guide to temperature.

Practical Advice

Fevers can be distressing for parents as well as their children. Try to remain calm and be reassuring. Stay with your child as much as possible, perhaps reading him books and stories. Many children regress when they are ill and need to be indulged for a short while.

Naturopathy

* Give plenty of fluids or sips of water at frequent intervals to avoid any risk of dehydration. Mineral water, lemon and honey or diluted fresh fruit juices, warmed or cold, are best. Carrot juice is a good choice for feverish children.
* Breastmilk is ideal for a nursing baby and may even enhance his resistance to the infection.
* Older babies or children who are reluctant to drink may suck ice cubes, a sponge or a flannel.
* Sponge your child down with tepid water if he is uncomfortably hot and sweaty or if the fever goes above 103/104°F (40°C).
* Apply a cool compress (a flannel soaked in cold water and squeezed out will do) to the forehead and lower back. Repeat when the flannel gets warm.
* Remove all extra clothing and bedding, then cover with a light cotton sheet. Don't mistake shivering for a sign that your child is cold – the body is simply trying to get rid of the fever. As his temperature cools, the shivering will stop.
* Most children with a fever are not hungry. Fasting with fluids for a day or two is fine as it allows the body to channel its energy reserves into fighting the infection and focus on recovery. Fevers can be exhausting, so build strength afterwards with plain

nutritious foods – vegetable soups, lightly buttered wholemeal toast, rice, fresh fruits and natural 'live' yoghurt.

Other Helpful Remedies

Herbal Remedy

* Infusions of Elderflower, Peppermint and Catnip are refreshing and help the body to throw off toxic wastes.

Aromatherapy

* For children over 6 months old: add cooling Lavender, Eucalyptus or Tea Tree essence to some sponging down water. These oils can also be added to tepid baths, providing your child does not drink from the bath water.

Homoeopathy

* Belladonna is the number one remedy for high fevers. Complaints will come on suddenly and be accompanied by burning red and hot flesh, throbbing and violent pain. The pulse will be rapid, eyes glassy and pupils dilated. Your child may be angry, delirious and thirsty, craving lemonade. Better for lying down. Worse for touch, jarring movements, and at around 3 p.m.

* Aconite is helpful in the early stages of any illness. For sudden onset of symptoms with high fever after exposure to cold, dry weather. Your child will be very restless, anxious, fearful, dry, hot and thirsty. Worse around midnight.

Give the 6c potency every 15 minutes for 4 doses.

Flower Remedies

* Five Flower Remedy (Healing Herbs) and Rescue Remedy (Bach Flower Remedies) are helpful if there is fearfulness and when the fever is a result of shock.

Biochemic Tissue Salts

* Ferr phos 3 times daily.

Chinese Medicine

Massage the Large Intestine 4 acupressure point – *see Figure 1, page 13*.

Doctor's Prescription

Paracetamol solution is generally recommended and can be given every 4 hours. This works by resetting the brain's temperature and helps the child feel more comfortable with the other symptoms. It does not make the illness go away any faster than it normally would, however.

Doctors do not recommend aspirin for children under 12 years old.

Seek help if a newborn baby gets a fever (fevers are uncommon in babies under 3 months old); consult your doctor. Feverish babies under 1 month of age may need to be hospitalized while the cause it found. A temperature higher than 105°F (40.5°C) is a cause for concern as your child may have a serious bacterial temperature. When the temperature exceeds 106°F (41°C) the majority of children have a serious illness such as pneumonia. In extreme cases a fever can lead to a fit. An older baby with a fever over 104°F which does not respond to sponging and natural remedies within 24 hours also needs specialist attention. If

your family has a history of convulsions accompanying fevers, if your baby or child refuses to drink, is listless and limp, difficult to awaken, won't stop crying or cries when touched or moved, is vague and confused or delirious, has trouble breathing or difficulty swallowing, has a rash with deep red or purplish spots, has a stiff neck or starts to twitch, these may be indicative of a serious illness such as pneumonia or meningitis. Seek medical help immediately.

FLU *See* **Influenza**

FOOD ALLERGIES

These are abnormal reactions to everyday foods in our diet. True food allergies are characterized by swelling of the face and shortness of breath within 30 minutes of eating the food; they are rare but can be fatal. Allergies to a particular food are highly individual, although foods most likely to cause such problems include strawberries, shellfish and peanuts.

Intolerances to foods are much more common and seem to becoming an increasing health problem. A sensitivity to certain foods often occurs in babies and children whose digestive systems are unable to cope with particular foods. Some believe that mass consumption of processed foods and weakened immune systems are largely responsible for causing food intolerances.

Symptoms are diverse and it is not always easy to recognize which particular food is the culprit. Ironically, foods that cause problems are often craved by the sufferer, so for instance your child may want to eat nothing but milk and ice-cream when he has in fact a sensitivity to cow's milk.

Typical Symptoms

Stomach cramps or colic, nausea, sickness and diarrhoea, a bloated stomach, headaches, skin irritations, hyperactivity, mood swings, fatigue and food cravings. Rarely, there may be an extreme reaction to a particular food resulting in swelling of the face, nose and throat, which can lead to breathing difficulties. This requires urgent medical attention.

If your child has experienced an acute reaction to peanuts or strawberries the solution is simply to make sure he does not eat them again. This will involve scrutinizing food labels and alerting all those who care for your child to the genuine problem of food allergy.

Food intolerances are much harder to identify and it is not a good idea to remove too many foods from your child's diet in the hopes of relieving symptoms. Limiting the diet can lead to nutritional deficiencies which may potentiate the problem in a child who is already quite finicky about eating.

Prevention is the best approach. Food allergies/intolerances can sometimes develop when a child is weaned too early. Ideally, breastfeed for at least the first 6 months of life and introduce first foods no earlier than 4 months of age. The best time is probably at around 5 to 6 months of age.

Try new foods slowly and cautiously, ensuring baby has adapted to each new one before moving on to the next. Start with simple fruit and vegetable purées, baby rice and millet.

Avoid giving milk and milk derivatives in the first year. Wheat products should also be limited, as this grain can often give rise to problems.

Diet and Nutritional Therapy

Many allergy sufferers improve when they are introduced to the basic Naturopathic diet.

Identifying and eliminating specific foods is best supervised by a qualified nutritionist. Kinesiology or muscle testing may be helpful in pinpointing problem foods too, but it should be done by a professional.

If you do remove a food such as cow's milk from your child's diet you will also have to eliminate all products containing it such as yoghurt, cheese, cream and skimmed milk before you will see any benefits. You will need to replace these with substitutes such as goat's, sheep's or soya milk. It may take up to 2 weeks for symptoms to clear. If this food really is the culprit the symptoms will recur whenever it is eaten again. However, you may find that after 6 to 12 months your child's tolerance resumes and small amounts can be taken again without provoking symptoms.

Food intolerances may be linked to nutritional deficiencies. It is important to give your child a wholesome and varied diet to ensure he gets all the nutrients needed to prevent intolerances from occurring. The mineral zinc is commonly lacking in people who suffer from food intolerances. A daily broad-spectrum vitamin and mineral supplement can help to prevent food intolerances and restore the health of sufferers.

Supplementing the diet with Evening Primrose Oil can reduce food intolerance symptoms. Fish oils may also be helpful.

Almond Milk Recipe

2–4 oz/60–120 g fresh blanched almonds
4–5 fl oz/120–150 ml fresh filtered or mineral water
full teaspoon of honey
pinch of sea salt

Put all the ingredients in a good processor or blender and mix until liquid. Strain the mixture to remove any remaining nuts. Do not use this recipe with newborn or very young children without first consulting a practitioner.

Other Helpful Remedies

Reflexology

Apply pressure to the adrenal gland reflex area on the hands and feet (*see Figure 2, page 53*).

Professional Therapy

Homoeopathy

A qualified homoeopath will aim to boost general immunity and so reduce the sensitivity to potential allergens.

Doctor's Prescription

Many food allergies are transient. Exclusion diets are best undertaken with the help of a nutritionist.

See also **Allergies**

H

HAY FEVER

Often known as seasonal rhinitis, this is an allergic response to pollens produced by blossoming flowers and ripening grasses.

Hay fever is not common in babies. It tends to occur later in childhood, between the ages of six and ten.

A predisposition towards hay fever usually runs in families with a history of asthma and eczema.

Hay fever is becoming increasingly common and it is now estimated that 1 in 10 people suffer from this problem.

In hay fever sufferers the immune system, which defends the body against invasion by bacteria and viruses, reacts abnormally to innocuous pollen grains in the atmosphere. When these grains make contact with the membranes lining the nose, throat and lungs, the body produces antibodies of the IgE variety. These latch on to special cells in the blood and tissues, which respond by pouring out inflammatory chemicals including the irritant, histamine, responsible for producing the classic hay fever symptoms.

Typical Symptoms

Violent sneezing, swollen and itchy eyes, snuffly and streaming nose, sore throat, skin rashes and stomach upsets. Hay fever sufferers may also become irritable, morose, have difficulty concentrating and feel fatigued.

In summer the most common troublemakers are the grass and nettle pollens released into the air in June and July. Sufferers who start sneezing before then may be reacting to certain tree pollens such as silver birch and horse-chestnut. Experts warn that the less colourful or showy plants, particularly weeds, often cause the most problems because their pollen grains are small and readily penetrate the nose, throat and lungs. Some people also react to mould spores which are released in damp weather.

The pollen count, recorded as 'grains per cubic metre', gives a rough guide as to your risk of having an allergic attack. Symptoms are often sparked off when the count reaches 50 and over.

The most effective treatment lies in avoiding the allergens as much as possible and boosting the body's natural resilience.

Preventative Measures

Keep your child away from fields and parks on dry, breezy, pollen-laden days. Pollen counts often soar in the early evening, so this is the time to stay inside.

Putting a net curtain over windows and wearing sunglasses helps to reduce pollen exposure.

Invest in an electronic air filter/ionizer for your child's bedroom as it will help to remove pollen, dust and other airborne irritants from the atmosphere.

The coast is a good refuge for hay fever sufferers, as the wind coming off the sea virtually eliminates pollen.

Hay fever sufferers often react to feathers, dust and house mites too. Invest in non-allergic bedding for your child, and damp dust his bedroom at least once a week.

Diet and Nutritional Therapy

* Cow's milk and other dairy products are best removed from the diet, especially during the hay fever season. They may be tolerated better during the winter months. Opt for alternatives such as goat's and sheep's milk, soya, almond or rice milk (*see page 159 for a recipe for Almond Milk*).

* Provide plenty of fresh fruits and vegetables. Add garlic to dishes, as this is reputedly helpful for hay fever sufferers.

* During a hay fever attack, give your child freshly squeezed lemon juice and water sweetened with honey to sip. This will help to soothe symptoms.

* Giving 500 mg of vitamin C with bioflavonoids (250 mg for under-threes) at the first sneeze can help to prevent a full-blown allergic reaction. Vitamin C acts like a natural anti-histamine.

* Pollen supplements may help to build up a tolerance to pollens in the environment. They must be taken at least a month before the start of the hay fever season. Start by giving a tiny crumb of pollen and build up to 1 teaspoon a day.

Hydrotherapy/Naturopathy

* Splash the face and immerse nostrils in cold water, as this helps to flush away pollen and dust particles.

* If your child is very congested you could try giving him a simple steam inhalation.

* For relieving swollen, itchy eyes, make a cooling eye mask by wrapping crushed ice in a flannel. You could also bathe the eyes with tepid salty water or an infusion of the herb Eyebright.

* Steep 1 oz/30 g of herb in 1 pint (600 ml) of boiling water for 10 minutes, strain and use as an eye bath when cool. Five to ten drops of Eyebright tincture in boiling water left to cool can also be used.

Other Helpful Remedies

Aromatherapy

* Chamomile and Peppermint essential oils can be beneficial when inhaled. For best effects, add a few drops to a vaporizer in your child's bedroom and use in the bath.

Chinese Medicine

* Add from 5 drops of Ma Huang tincture to 1 cup (240 ml) of boiling water. Let it cool down and give as sips.

Biochemic Tissue Salts

* Combination H: 2 tablets every hour.

Reflexology

Work the adrenal gland reflex area on the feet and hands (*see Figure 2, page 53*).

Herbal Remedies

* Herbalists may recommend giving Plantain tea.

* Immune Balance Formula (*see page 32*) may help to calm an over-reactive immune system: 10 drops in 6 fl oz/180 ml of water 3 times a day.

Homoeopathy

There are numerous remedies for hay fever symptoms; the following ones are most commonly recommended.

* Allium cepa – for burning, smarting eyes, a streaming and stuffy nose, tickling in the back of the throat. Eyes sensitive to light. Symptoms better in open air.

* Arsenicum album – burning eyelids and bloodshot eyes that are gritty and sensitive to light. Watery and burning nasal discharge, burning throat, wheezing. Sufferer feels restless, worried and exhausted by symptoms.

* Arundo – itching in the nostrils, ears and roof of the mouth.

* Euphrasia – swollen, burning eyes with thick discharge, streaming nose, cough with phlegm. Symptoms worse indoors.

* Gelsemium – heavy swollen eyes, sneezing and streaming nose, sore throat. Sufferer feels apathetic, listless, giddy and trembling.

* Nat mur – smarting, light-sensitive eyes that feel bruised, violent sneezing, watery discharge from nose.

Cough which makes the eyes water more. Sufferer feels depressed and touchy.

Give the 6C potency, one dose every 2 hours for up to 4 doses.

Note: Treatment is particularly successful when a constitutional remedy is prescribed by a professional homoeopathic practitioner.

Doctor's Prescription

Treatment aims at dampening down the inflammatory reactions. Anti-histamines are generally recommended. Sometimes inhaled medications including steroids can reverse and control hay fever symptoms.

New research is looking at preventing the reaction between the antibody and allergen, which causes the inflammation.

See also **Allergies**

HEADACHES

There are many different reasons for headaches. They are often a sign of anxiety and general stress. Headaches may accompany a cold, fever, or infectious illness. A headache may also be a reaction to hunger, too much sleep, noise or weather changes.

Dull throbbing headaches with feelings of nausea may be a symptom of an allergy or food intolerance. Recurrent headaches are often linked to poor posture and are related to excessive tension in the neck and shoulder muscles.

Practical Advice

If your child suffers from headaches quite regularly, look for a pattern of recurrence. Do they always come on after your child eats a certain type of food or when he is colouring (volatile chemicals in felt tip pens can cause allergic reactions)?

Try these preventative measures:

* Give regular meals including a good breakfast.

* Make sure your child gets enough sleep and encourage a nap after lunch.

* Encourage plenty of fresh air and exercise outdoors. A short walk can work wonders for clearing the head.

Homoeopathy

* Aconite – for sudden violent headaches that come on after a fright, shock or getting chilled.

* Belladonna – for throbbing, hammering headaches in the back of the head, eyes, forehead and temples that come on suddenly. Worse for cold, heat, light, bending down, walking and at around 3 p.m. Better for resting the head and lying down in a quiet, darkened room.

* Gelsemium – head feels heavy, pain in the back of the head spreading to the forehead. Develops gradually, coming on after weather changes or with flu.

* Mag phos – known as homoeopathic aspirin. It is useful for relieving headaches in sensitive, nervous people who often talk about their pains. Better for heat, firm pressure. Worse for cold, uncovering, touch. Very effective when crushed and sipped in some still mineral or spring water.

* Nat mur – for migraine-type headache.

Give the 6C potency every 30 minutes for up to 4 doses. Repeat if needed.

Aromatherapy and Massage

* For children over 1 year old: Chamomile, Lavender, Eucalyptus and Peppermint in a base of Grapeseed oil.

* For children over 5 years old: you can also use Marjoram and Rosemary.

* For children over 7 years old: you can also use Melissa and Basil, combining any two of the recommended essences together: a total of 8 to 12 drops in 30 ml of Grapeseed oil.

Stroke your child across his forehead with your fingertips, applying a light pressure with your forefinger to his temples and holding for a minute. Stroke down the back of his neck and across his shoulders.

Other Helpful Remedies

Herbal Remedy

* Peppermint tisane is refreshing and helps clear the head. It also aids digestion and may ease food-related headaches.

Chinese Medicine

* Traditionally, Chrysanthemum is given for headaches. Make a mild tisane by infusing a teaspoon of petals in 1 cup (240 ml) of boiling water and steep for 5 minutes. Sweeten to taste.

* The benefits are enhanced by working the Triple Warmer 23 and Gall Bladder 1 acupressure points (*see Figure 1, page 13*).

Biochemic Tissue Salts

* Kali phos or Nat sulph: 2 tablets every hour until symptoms clear.

Reflexology

Work the head and solar plexus reflex areas on the feet and hands (*see Figure 2, page 53*).

Professional Therapies

Osteopathy

Can be helpful if your child experiences recurrent headaches from an early age. Headaches may be related to spinal misalignment and muscular tensions originating from birth or from falls and seemingly minor injuries.

Homoeopathy

A professional homoeopath will consider headaches in the context of a whole symptom profile.

Doctor's Prescription

Headaches are often anxiety-related and your doctor may ask you to observe the pattern of the headaches: for example, do they occur at weekends and holidays or only during term-time? Migraine can occur in childhood and may also present as abdominal pain. Painkillers or preventative tablets may be necessary, but most headaches resolve with time and reassurance.

Seek help if your child complains of persistent headaches which have no obvious cause or headaches which come and go in sudden attacks.

See also **Allergies, Food Allergies**

HICCUPS

Hiccups are due to a sudden contraction of the diaphragm which allows air to rush into the lungs. Some babies hiccup a lot, even while they are in the uterus. Babies may hiccup every time they feed, laugh or get excited. In childhood, hiccups may result from stomach problems or after eating certain foods such as onions or peppers.

Hiccups are not usually serious and tend to stop as suddenly as they begin. Here are a few remedies that may be worth trying.

* Mag phos (Biochemic tissue salts): 2 tablets straight away, repeating after an hour if necessary.

* Give your child a glass of water to drink 'upside down', i.e. tipping his head forwards and sipping from the other side of the glass.

* Get your child to breathe into a paper bag.

* Give him a wedge of lemon to suck.

* For babies, give water sweetened with honey on a spoon.

* Put a drop of Mandarin essential oil on a tissue for your child to inhale.

Seek help when hiccups are prolonged and exhausting. Occasionally hiccups can be dangerous, so it is worth checking with your doctor if your child suffers from repeated attacks of violent hiccuping.

HIVES

Also known as urticaria or nettle rash, this is a skin condition characterized by itchy white lumps or weals with a red inflamed area around them. Hives are usually triggered by an allergic reaction to certain foods, additives, drugs (particularly aspirin), insect bites or even stress.

Prevention is the best approach. Try to find out what is causing the reaction and try to make sure your child avoids contact with whatever it is.

Common food triggers are strawberries, shellfish, tomatoes, red currants, chocolate, eggs, wheat, cow's milk and food additives. You could try excluding each food, one at a time, for a week or two to see if symptoms are relieved.

Hydrotherapy/Naturopathy

* Add 3 tablespoons of sodium bicarbonate to the bath to relieve itching.

* Add 5 tablespoons of oatmeal to the bath to soothe the rash.

Homoeopathy

* Apis mel – for burning and stinging, red and itching rash with swelling.

* Arsenicum – swelling with burning pain, vomiting and diarrhoea.

* Rhus tox – burning, itching, stinging rash; worse for cold and after scratching. Often accompanied by aching pains in the joints.

* Urtica urens – for stinging, itchy rashes especially if triggered by shellfish.

Give the 6c potency 3 times a day. Continue as necessary.

Other Helpful Remedies

Herbal Remedies

* Apply soothing Aloe Vera gel to the affected area.

Chinese Medicine

* Caltrop fruit tincture diluted in water can be used to bathe the affected area.

Doctor's Prescription

Anti-histamine cream or tablets may be recommended.

HYPERACTIVITY

Hyperactivity is defined as abnormally overactive and restless behaviour. Children affected by this condition can range from being a bit of a handful to aggressive, violent and extremely difficult to live with.

Typical Symptoms

Constantly on the go, quick thinking, irritable, has difficulty concentrating or settling down to anything for any length of time, cries and shouts a great deal, throws tantrums frequently, does not sleep well and is a finicky eater.

Babies will be fidgety and cry incessantly, feed poorly and often have eczema. At school, hyperactive children are disruptive and tend to have learning disabilities.

Not many children are truly hyperactive, they are just extremely energetic. It has been said that even an ultra-fit athlete would feel exhausted by bedtime after following a toddler around all day.

Between 2 and 5 per cent of children, and 10 times as many boys as girls, are estimated to be seriously hyperactive. Nevertheless, this condition has become increasingly prevalent in the last decade and is still a growing concern. Dealing with such a child can be stressful and exhausting. Fortunately, hyperactive children often respond very well to a natural approach to treatment, becoming far more manageable and fun to live with.

Naturopathy

Naturopaths and nutritionists alike feel that hyperactivity is largely diet-related. Behavioural problems may be triggered by specific food intolerances – often to milk, wheat and eggs, sensitivities to natural and artificial chemicals (red and orange colourings most frequently cause problems) and nutritional deficiencies.

As so many different foods have been implicated in hyperactivity it is essential to seek professional nutritional advice before radically altering your child's diet. However, simply switching to a diet based on natural ingredients and avoiding all junk and processed foods often brings behavioural improvements.

Choose a strictly wholefood diet that includes plenty of fish, poultry, cereals, fruits and vegetables, except those suspected of causing problems. Avoid giving sugar in any form (that is, as sweets, biscuits, cakes or fizzy drinks).

The Feingold Diet

Dr Ben F. Feingold has carried out extensive and successful work with hyperactive and learning disabled children. His diet eliminates two main food groups:

* Group 1: all foods with artificial colours and flavours, along with the preservatives BHA and BHT

* Group 2: fruits and vegetables containing natural salicylates. These include almonds, apples, apricots, cherries,

berries, grapes, raisins, green peppers, oranges, peaches, peas and tomatoes.

Give supplements of Evening Primrose oil (3 × 500 mg) and Cod liver oil (2 ml a day) for 6 to 8 weeks. The contents of these capsules could be added to a night-time bottle or mug of milk.

The Hyperactive Children's Support Group, founded by Vicky Colquhoun and Sally Bunday, has found that hyperactive children tend to be deficient in four essential fatty acids normally found in foods such as eggs and fish. Signs of such deficiency include excessive thirst, dry skin and allergies. Their work has been supported by a major study published in the *American Journal of Clinical Nutrition*, which found that 40 per cent of hyperactive children were deficient in these essential fatty acids.

All four essential fatty acids are supplied by a combination of Evening Primrose and Cod liver oil.

Any active child has higher requirements for all nutrients. Low levels of certain nutrients are common in children suffering from hyperactivity. These tend to be the B complex vitamins, especially B_1 and B_6, as well as the minerals calcium, magnesium and zinc.

Give your child bottled mineral water to drink, as tap water can contain chemicals which may trigger hyperactivity. As bottled mineral water can be expensive, a cheaper alternative would be to purchase a jug filter to remove some of the impurities in tap water.

Aspirin and artificial flavours in vitamin pills may provoke hyperactivity. Remember, many children's medicines have artificial colours and flavourings.

Massage and Aromatherapy

Massage is a good way of calming an agitated child – if you can catch him! Massaging either the hands or feet is an ideal way to begin. After a while you may be able to include the shoulders and back.

* Chamomile helps to soothe the nervous system. Add the appropriate number of drops (*see page 6*) to your chosen carrier oil. The essence could also be added to the bath.

Other Helpful Remedies

Herbal Remedies

* Add up to 15 drops of Chamomile tincture to a glass of water or small bottle of milk. This is an extremely safe way of soothing a restless baby or child.

* Happy Child Formula (*see page 33*): 10 drops in 6 fl oz/180 ml water 3 times a day. For restless babies, add 5 drops to a small bottle of milk.

A professional herbal practitioner can prescribe other herbal sedatives which are safe and non-addictive.

Flower Remedies

* Black Eyed Susan (Australian Bush Essences) – for those who are always on the go, rushing, constantly striving and impatient.

* Impatiens (Bach Flower Remedies/Healing Herbs) – for impatient, impulsive people who dislike restraints and are prone to nervous tension, over-exertion and accidents, temper outbursts, irritability and indigestion.

* Jacaranda (Australian Bush Essences) – for those who are changeable, scattered, always rushing around and accident-prone.

Reflexology

Apply pressure to the adrenal gland reflex area on the feet and hands (*see Figure 2, page 53*).

Professional Therapies

Homoeopathy

A professional homoeopath should be consulted if you are considering giving your child homoeopathic remedies for hyperactivity.

Osteopathy

Cranial osteopathy as part of a complete osteopathic assessment and treatment can be helpful in some cases of hyperactivity.

Diet and Nutritional Therapy

A professional nutritionist should be consulted if you are considering any kind of exclusion diet and to help prescribe corrective supplements.

Doctor's Prescription

Stimulant drugs such as amphetamines may be given to motivate the part of the brain which suppresses excess activity. These drugs also suppress the appetite and may cause nausea and abdominal pain.

Psychotherapy and assessment for special educational needs may be necessary.

Severely hyperactive children may be given the controversial amphetamine-type drug Ritalin (methylphanidate), which improves mental functioning. Little is known of its long-term effects. It is only considered when lack of concentration and attention are disabling and after psychological treatments have failed.

See also **Behavioural Problems**

I

IMMUNIZATIONS *See* **Vaccinations**

IMPETIGO

This highly contagious bacterial skin infection is quite common. It can be caused by an infected scratch or insect bite, or caught from other children with the condition. It commonly occurs after a cold when the natural defences are weak. Eczema-prone children are particularly susceptible.

The condition will not go away of its own accord and sores must be treated the moment they are noticed.

Typical Symptoms

Bright red spots or sores, which usually appear first on the face. These turn into pustules, containing yellow pus, which crust over.

The rash may spread from the face down to the chest and lower body.

Practical Advice

Impetigo is contagious, so change your child's linen daily and do not share towels, flannels and bedding. These should be boil washed until the condition clears.

Discourage scratching, as this allows the sores to spread.

Aromatherapy

* Add 5 drops of Tea Tree oil to a small bowl of boiled water and wash the sores thoroughly using clean cotton wool for each sore.

* Apply a compress to the affected area. You will need a piece of lint cut into a rectangle large enough to cover the area of the sore twice over. Soak the lint in diluted Tea Tree oil and bandage the body. Leave for an hour, then remove so the area is exposed. Repeat this treatment until the sores disappear.

Herbal Remedies

* Bathe the sores with Marigold solution 3 times a day. Add 5 drops of Marigold tincture to a $1/2$ pint (300 ml) of cooled, boiled water.

* Dab Calendula cream or ointment onto the sores in between bathing and at night-time.

* To strengthen the immune system, give 5–15 drops of

Echinacea tincture in cooled, boiled water or fruit juice daily.

Homeopathy

* Ant crud – for oozing eruptions with thick, yellow crusts. Worse on the face; individual sores join together. Looks worse after bathing.

* Graphites – for scabby, oozing eruptions with sticky discharge.

* Merc sol – for deep, open sores with yellowish crusts exuding offensive-smelling pus.

* Rhus tox – for extremely itchy and burning sores, with blister-like eruptions.

Give 3 doses of the 6C potency and repeat for the next 4 days if there is some improvement. If there is no relief of symptoms, consult a professional homoeopath.

Doctor's Prescription

Antibiotics are given to kill the staphylococcus bacteria which causes impetigo.

INFECTIONS

Infections are caused by bacteria, viruses and fungi when they invade and spread through the body. Symptoms are the body's way of responding to their presence and, while different pathogens tend to produce different patterns of illness, certain symptoms are characteristic of most infections.

Typical Symptoms

Fever, inflammation, swollen glands, aching joints, redness and pus.

How the Immune System Works

Every day we come in contact with countless different viruses and bacteria. Protection is provided by a highly effective fighting force, the immune system, which defends us against unwanted invaders.

Viruses and bacteria are unable to do any damage unless they can enter body tissues in the first place. The primary line of defence is provided by mucous membranes lining the lungs, nasal passages, intestines and all openings of the body. Healthy membranes are continually washed with a thin mucus enriched with protective substances such as the enzyme lysozyme, which is capable of instantly destroying these pathogens.

If this protective barrier is breached, the main part of the immune system comes into play. The main defenders are called T and B lymphocytes (white blood cells), which are produced in the lymph glands and spleen. The T lymphocytes are capable of recognizing foreign invaders – an attribute given them by the thymus gland, which orchestrates the whole immune system. These T cells recruit the help of B cells and are themselves capable of releasing deadly chemicals that attack the invader.

The B cells make antibodies which act rather like strait-jackets, immobilizing the invader until it can be dealt with. The B cells can also 'remember' what kind of antibody it needs to make if the same virus or bacteria invades again.

Mothers endow their newborn babies with a temporary immunity to infections. This protection takes the form of antibodies to bacteria or viruses which the mother's immune system has encountered in the past. These antibodies are passed to the baby via the placenta. The colostrum in breastmilk adds to this immunity. Previously it was thought that this natural protection lasted for about the first three months of life, but recent studies suggest that fully breastfed babies (that is, those breastfed for six months or longer) are protected right up until their own immune systems are well established.

Strengthening the Natural Defences

Natural therapists believe that a healthy diet, plenty of fresh air and exercise, sound sleep and a happy disposition are your child's best defences against infections. Naturopaths in particular view harmful bacteria and viruses as opportunistic, that is, only invading if the conditions are right. Emphasis is placed on creating a healthy environment which potential pathogens will find uninviting.

Children prone to recurrent infections can be helped by natural remedies which aim to fortify and strengthen the natural defence system.

Diet and Nutritional Therapy

During an infection the body's requirement for all nutrients escalates. Certain vitamins and minerals in particular play an important role in supporting the immune system.

* Vitamin A – helps to prevent infections by protecting the mucus membranes. When vitamin A is undersupplied, the cells of the mucous membranes become dry and can no longer secrete mucous or produce bacteria-digesting enzymes. Research indicates that during an infection vitamin A should be immediately increased. Some nutritionists recommend giving 25,000 iu for a few days or while the infection lasts (no longer than one week).

* Vitamin A can be toxic in excess so never give more than 5,000 iu daily on a regular basis.

   Natural sources are the best way to keep vitamin A levels topped up. Green- and orange-coloured vegetables are rich in beta-carotene, a safe substance the body readily converts to vitamin A.

* Vitamin C – can help to prevent and fight infections in many ways: by inhibiting the growth of bacteria, aiding the production of antibodies and making bacterial and viral toxins harmless.

  This nutrient is most effective when given at the onset of an infection or the first moment symptoms appear.

* Give 500 mg to 1 g (half this amount for under-threes), 3 times a day for 2 days. Good natural sources are blackcurrants, parsley, broccoli, green peppers, strawberries, oranges and tomatoes.

* Vitamin E works alongside vitamins A and C in neutralizing free radicals, the harmful substances generated during an infection. Good natural sources are wheatgerm, seeds and seed oils, margarine and egg yolk.

* Vitamins B_6 (pyridoxine) and B_5 (pantothenic acid) are needed for producing antibodies. A lack of these nutrients predisposes us towards continuous colds and respiratory infections.

* The mineral zinc has a profound influence on immune responses; low levels are linked to recurrent infections. Good natural sources are liver, lean red meat, poultry, cheddar cheese, beans and lentils.

* Iron – lack of this mineral is associated with a low resistance to infections. Children are susceptible to iron deficiency. (Natural sources of iron are listed on page 24.)

Herbal Remedies

* Echinacea (Purple Coneflower) – studies have found that this colourful flower has a stimulatory and regulatory effect on the immune system. Extracts have anti-viral properties and are especially effective against influenza and herpes.

* Children's Immune Formula (*see page 32*) is also helpful: 10 drops in 6 fl oz/180 ml water 3 times a day. For babies over 3 months old: 5 drops in a small bottle of milk.

* Bee propolis is a concentrated source of 'dihydroflavonoids', substances with powerful anti-viral, anti-bacterial, anti-inflammatory and antioxidant properties. Given as a supplement, especially during the winter months, it can help enhance the immune system and ward off coughs and colds.

Other Helpful Remedies

Homoeopathy

* Aconite can help to nip infections in the bud. Give 1 dose of the 30C potency in the early stages of colds, fevers and inflammations.

Aromatherapy

All essential oils are natural antiseptics; certain ones such as Tea Tree and Eucalyptus have anti-viral, anti-bacterial and anti-fungal properties. Add a few drops to your child's baths to keep his immune system healthy and protect him from the endless round of infectious illnesses that circulate in nurseries and schools. Tea Tree and Eucalyptus can also be sprayed throughout the house or used in vaporizers for added protection if anyone in the family has an infectious illness.

Reflexology

Work the immune system reflex areas on the hands and feet (*see Figure 2, page 53*).

Relaxation

A sudden shock and/or lingering stress weakens the body's immunity to infections. A child who is tense, worried or anxious is more likely to catch frequent colds, coughs, and so forth – so try to find ways to combat stress in your child's life.

Professional Therapy

Osteopathy

Osteopathy balances the entire body framework so that every organ and part of the body, including the immune system, functions more efficiently. Treatment can often help to strengthen the resilience of children prone to recurrent infections.

Homoeopathy

A professional homoeopath will aim to strengthen your child's natural resistance and so reduce the frequency of recurrent infections with an appropriate constitutional remedy.

Doctor's Prescription

Most doctors are reluctant to prescribe antibiotics unless absolutely necessary, as these drugs have been over-used in the Western world and some bacteria have developed resistance to them. Many coughs, colds and sore throats are caused by viruses and will not, therefore, respond to such antibiotics. If infections persist, you should consult your doctor.

INFLUENZA

Commonly called flu, this is an acute infection of the respiratory tract, similar to a cold but far more severe.

Typical Symptoms

Sore throat, runny or congested nose, cough, fever, headache, aching limbs, nausea and weakness.

Influenza is caused by viruses of many different strains; new ones tend to appear each winter leading to widespread epidemics.

A dose of flu normally lasts between two and five days. Bedrest is essential when symptoms are at their worst. It is also important to allow plenty of time for convalescence otherwise flu can leave your child feeling debilitated and depressed for many weeks afterwards.

Diet and Nutritional Therapy

* Although your child is unlikely to want to eat, it is a good idea to sustain nourishment with plenty of freshly squeezed fruit and vegetable juices diluted with water. Try to tempt him with delicious blends such as carrot and apple, grape and kiwi fruit, tangerine and papaya. Limit to 5 fl oz (150 ml) of each juice blend a day.

* Give hot apple and cinnamon tea to sip (*see* **Colds** for recipe).

* Vitamin C will help to fight the infection. Give 500 mg 3 times a day (half this dose for children under 3).

* During recovery it is important to build up zinc reserves, as this mineral supports the immune system.

Herbal Remedies

* Echinacea will help to fight off the flu virus and revitalize the immune system. Use 5 to 10 drops of tincture in fruit juice or mineral water.
* Children's Immunity Formula (*see page 32*) will help to strengthen your child's immune defences.
* A combination of Elderflower and Peppermint is good for relieving the symptoms of flu. Ideally, give herbal teas every hour or two, interspersed with diluted fruit juices or hot lemon and honey drinks.

Other Helpful Remedies

Homoeopathy

* Gelsemium is the first choice of remedy for flu, especially if there is shivering up and down the spine, aching muscles and a feeling of heaviness in the head and eyes. Give Gelsemium 6C every hour for 3 doses. Repeat if needed.

Aromatherapy

Eucalyptus can help to ease congestion. Sprinkle a few drops onto a tissue and tuck into your child's pillow, or place a few drops in a bowl of steaming water in the bedroom. For children over 5 try a steam inhalation: add 2–3 drops of Eucalyptus in a basin of steaming hot water, cover the head with a towel and encourage deep breathing through the nose. Always supervise your child during a steam inhalation treatment.

Biochemic Tissue Salts

* Nat sulph: 2 tablets 3 times a day.

INSOMNIA *See* **Sleeping Problems**

IRRITABILITY

Every baby and child is likely to be irritable from time to time. Irritability is often a sign of frustration that results from trying to crawl, walk, talk and so forth. Those who are adventurous, fearless individuals who want to push the boundaries faster than they should are liable to be particularly irritable when thwarted.

Irritability is only a problem when it becomes stressful to both child and parents. Some natural remedies have soothing properties and can help to restore a sense of calmness and emotional balance.

Homoeopathy

* Chamomilla – for irritable, angry babies, especially when teething. Babies who need this remedy will whine, scream and reject attempts at being comforted, often becoming spiteful towards their parents. They will insist on being carried.

* Lycopodium – for babies who are irritable after a sleep and are often cross all day; for toddlers who are irritable and dictatorial, having tantrums if contradicted. They will kick and scream after a nap or on waking in the morning.

* Rheum – for babies who are irritable, restless and difficult when teething.

Give the 30C potency once and watch for improvement. Repeat if the irritability returns.

Flower Remedies

* Black Eyed Susan (Australian Bush Essences) – for those who are always on the go, rushing, constantly striving and impatient.

* Chamomile (Flower Essence Society) – for those who are easily upset, irritable and moody, unable to release emotional tension, which leads to insomnia. Also good for children's stomach complaints.

* Impatiens (Bach Flower Remedies/Healing Herbs) – for impatient, impulsive children who dislike restraint and are quick to act and prone to irritability, temper outbursts and accidents.

Other Helpful Remedies

Aromatherapy

* Chamomile is renowned for soothing the nervous system. Add a few drops of Chamomile essential oil to a night-time bath, sprinkle onto your child's pillow case or tuck a tissue scented with this essence into baby's cot.

Herbal Remedy

* For irritable babies, you could also add a few drops of Chamomile tincture to an evening bottle of milk. For toddlers and older children, try sips of weak Chamomile tisane sweetened with honey.

Biochemic Tissue Salts

* Kali phos: 2 tablets every hour until the child seems calmer.

Professional Therapy

Osteopathy

Treatment focusing on the cranium can be helpful in some instances.

JAUNDICE (IN NEWBORNS)

Many babies develop a mild form of jaundice two to four days after birth. The skin has a golden, sun-tanned appearance and the eye whites have a yellowish tinge.

Newborn jaundice is due to the build-up of a yellow pigment in the blood (bilirubin) normally broken down by the liver. It occurs because the liver is not yet fully matured. Jaundice is more common in premature babies and in babies bruised during birth.

Jaundice can also recur as a result of rhesus incompatibility – for example, when a mother with rhesus negative blood gives birth to a rhesus-positive baby. Nowadays this problem is almost sure to be anticipated before the birth, and steps taken to minimize the consequences.

Some jaundiced babies become lethargic and feed less often, but the condition rarely causes complications unless there is a more serious underlying medical problem, which should be detected by your midwife or health visitor.

Practical Advice

Breastfeed your baby frequently. Plenty of fluids are needed to flush away the bilirubin.

Expose baby to sunlight as often as possible, but be wary of the dangers of sunburn on hot summer days. If it is chilly outdoors, make sure baby is bundled up well, exposing only his face to the sun's rays.

Homoeopathy

* Chelidonium majus is the main remedy for jaundice in babies, as it helps the liver to adjust to life outside the womb.
* If baby is otherwise well, give Chelidonium 6C, 1 dose every 2 hours for a day. If other symptoms are present it is a good idea to consult a professional homoeopath who can prescribe a more appropriate remedy.

Doctor's Prescription

If jaundice persists it should be investigated, as it may be caused by a narrowing of a duct in the liver or an inability of the liver to break down pigment due to a lack of enzymes.

L

LACTOSE INTOLERANCE

This is an inability to digest a sugar called lactose found in milk due to a lack of the digestive enzyme, lactase. Lactose intolerance tends to be inherited and is especially common in those of Asian, African and Mediterranean origins. The problem can also develop after a bout of gastro-enteritis. Children often grow out of this problem between the ages of 10 and 12.

Typical Symptoms

Bloating, excessive wind, stomach cramps or colic, vomiting, frothy diarrhoea. Often resembles colitis and may be mistaken for this.

Diet and Nutritional Therapy

If you suspect your baby or child may have difficulty digesting milk, exclude it for at least 2 weeks and see if the symptoms clear. Replace with soya, almond or rice milk (*see page 159 for a recipe for almond milk*).

As milk is an important source of calcium for young children, if you do exclude it from the diet be sure to give plenty of calcium-rich foods. Good natural sources are salmon and sardines, dark green leafy vegetables, peas, kidney beans, haricot beans, chickpeas, lentils, dried apricots and sesame seeds.

You can buy lactase, the enzyme responsible for digestive lactose, from healthfood stores. When added to milk and left overnight it digests the lactose so it no longer causes problems. It is also possible to buy lactose-reduced milk from most supermarkets.

See also **Food Allergies**

LARYNGITIS

Inflammation of the larynx or voice box generally caused by a viral or bacterial infection. It can also be caused by over-straining the voice. In children laryngitis may manifest as croup.

Typical Symptoms

Hoarseness, an irritating cough, dry sore throat and sometimes loss of voice. If voice loss lasts for more than a week, consult your doctor.

Naturopathy

* Salt water makes an excellent antiseptic gargle for easing laryngitis.

* A cold pack applied to the neck can help to reduce inflammation and soreness.
* Run a large handkerchief under the cold tap and place around the neck. Hold there until it warms up. Repeat.
* Steam inhalations can also help to soothe inflamed mucous membranes in the larynx for children over 5. To enhance the benefits add 1 drop of Chamomile and 1 drop of Lavender essential oils to the bowl of steaming water. Always supervise steam inhalations.

Other Helpful Remedies

Diet and Nutritional Therapy

* Include plenty of onions in the diet for their antiseptic properties.
* Apricots and bilberries are also reputed to ease laryngitis.
* Sipping freshly squeezed lemon juice in hot water sweetened with honey helps to relieve symptoms.

Herbal Remedies

* Echinacea helps the immune system to overcome the viral and bacterial infections responsible for laryngitis. At the first signs of symptoms add 5–15 drops of Echinacea tincture to boiling water. When cooled, give as sips.
* Elderflower Syrup (*see page 31*) is very soothing: 1 teaspoon 3 times a day.

Aromatherapy

* Lavender is useful for treating all infections of the respiratory tract. Add a few drops of essential oil to baths and massage Lavender diluted in Almond oil into the throat and chest area.
* You could also try making a tisane made from Lavender flowers. Infuse 1 oz/30 g of flowers and flowering tips in 2 pints/1 litre of boiling water for 5 minutes. Strain and give a cupful sweetened with honey 3 times a day.

Doctor's Prescription

Most cases resolve of their own accord. A course of antibiotics is usually tried for persistent symptoms.

LICE AND NITS

Head lice are tiny brownish-grey insects, slightly smaller than a match-head, that can live in the hair. They lay their minuscule cream-coloured eggs on hair shafts close to the scalp, where they become glued into position. When the baby lice hatch they leave their empty shells, known as nits, behind. These look rather like dandruff.

School children are particularly vulnerable as these parasites jump from one head to another. Frequent shampooing does not deter them, indeed lice actually seem to prefer clean hair. Vigorous brushing does, however, help to keep them away.

Look for signs of lice and nits under a fringe, by the nape of the neck or above the ears.

Typical Symptoms

The scalp feels itchy and can become inflamed. Itching does not usually occur until the lice have been present for a couple of months, so check the head regularly and nip them in the bud before things reach this stage.

Practical Advice

While treating the hair and scalp you should wash everything that comes in contact with the head – bedding, hats, scarves, headbands – with soap powder. Combs and brushes can be washed in a little special aromatherapy shampoo (*see below*).

Aromatherapy

As a deterrent, especially if there is an outbreak of lice at your child's nursery or school, wash the hair once a week with a shampoo containing the following essential oils:

* For children over 1 year old: 6 drops of Geranium to 30 ml of mild shampoo. Apply to dry hair and cover the head with a shower cap for 10 minutes. After rinsing thoroughly, rinse hair with 1 cup (240 ml) of water containing 2 drops of the same essence. Comb through with a fine-toothed comb.
* For children over 6 years old: use a blend of Geranium, Rosemary and Lemon, 3 drops of each essence to 30 ml of a mild shampoo and use in the same way as above.

If you suspect your child has lice and nits, massage the head thoroughly with a special scalp oil:

Headlice Recipe

* 10 drops Geranium

* 10 drops Rosemary
* 5 drops Lemon
* 5 drops Tea Tree

Add the essential oils to 50 ml of Almond or Grapeseed oil. Massage about 10 ml of this blend very thoroughly into the hair and scalp. Comb through, wrap the hair up in a dry towel and leave on for at least 2 hours, longer if possible, before shampooing out. Rinse with the appropriate aromatherapy hair rinse and comb hair with a fine-toothed comb. Repeat 2 days later, and again after 8 days to prevent re-infestation.

Other Helpful Remedies

Homoeopathy

* Psorinum 30C, one single dose, to children who are prone to recurrent infestations of lice.

Doctor's Prescription

Generally a shampoo or scalp lotion containing malathion, a mild pesticide, is recommended to kill the lice. As lice are notorious for developing immunity to certain preparations, new ones are brought into use roughly every six months. Consult your pharmacist to get the most up-to-date preparation. Concerns have also been raised recently about the possible over-use of preparations containing pesticides on young children.

M

MEASLES

A highly contagious disease caused by a potentially dangerous virus which generally occurs between 1 and 3 years of age. Babies under 8 months old rarely get measles because they have acquired passive immunity from their mothers.

Children need careful nursing through measles to reduce any possibility of complications. These include ear infections, respiratory problems, pneumonia and (rarely) inflammation of the brain or encephalitis, so always consult your doctor if your child develops the classic symptoms of measles.

Recovery should be complete after 10 days; an attack of measles usually confers life-long immunity.

Incubation period: 7 to 12 days.

Infectious period: from a few days before the rash appears until 5 days after it goes.

Measles

Typical Symptoms

Starts like a cold with a cough and sore, watery eyes.

A temperature develops and the child feels more unwell. Small spots like grains of sand (Koplik spots) may appear in the mouth, on the inside of the cheeks, before the characteristic rash appears a day or two later. A blotchy rash with raised spots usually begins behind the ears and spreads down the body. Other possible symptoms are headache, stomach pains, vomiting and diarrhoea; the eyes may be very sensitive to light.

Be resigned to caring for a measly baby or child for at least a week.

Keep a child with sore eyes out of bright light. The best place is bed with the curtains drawn and the lights dimmed. Watching television is not good for light-sensitive eyes.

Follow the general guidelines for **Childhood Diseases**; *see also* **Infections**.

Homoeopathy

Homoeopathy is especially helpful for relieving the cough and sore eyes that can accompany measles, as well as deterring the development of more serious complications.

* Aconite – for sudden onset of fever with a burning, itchy rash. Give the 6C potency, 1 dose every hour for up to 4 doses. Repeat if needed.
* Belladonna – when the sufferer is restless, flushed, has a high temperature and delirium, sore throat, is upset by noise, light and movement. Give 1 or 2 doses of the 30C potency.
* Byronia – if the rash is slow to appear and symptoms include by a painful, dry cough. The sufferer will be thirsty, irritable, worse for movement. Give 2 to 3

doses of the 6C or 30c potency.

See also Recipe under **Childhood Diseases**.

Herbal Remedies

* Echinacea will help to combat the virus and should be used once the fever has started to come down. Use up to 15 drops of Echinacea tincture in 1 cup (240 ml) of cooled boiled water.
* Eyebright herb will help to soothe sore, sensitive eyes. Make an infusion and, when cool, strain and use to bathe the eyes.
* Yarrow infusion helps to reduce a fever and should be given during the first stages of illness. Pour 1 cup (240 ml) of water over 1 teaspoon of herb, infuse for 15 minutes, strain and give 3 times a day.
* An infusion of Chickweed can be used to bathe the rash. Soak cotton wool in this and dab the skin, or add a cupful to the bath.

Other Helpful Remedies

Aromatherapy

* Chamomile and Lavender will help to relieve the rash and aid recovery. Add 5 drops of each to a small bowl containing tepid water to make a sponging-down solution. Soak your sponge or flannel in this solution, wring out and gently dab over the whole body.
* Add these essences to the bath, using the appropriate number of drops depending on age (*see page 6*).

Hydrotherapy

Warm baths with 3 tablespoons of baking soda will soothe the rash as well as being generally therapeutic.

Professional Therapy

Homoeopathy

While a homoeopath will generally consider it more beneficial for a child to have measles and establish a natural immunity to this disease, in some instances they can give Moribillinum 30C as a preventative measure during a measles epidemic.

Doctor's Prescription

Antibiotics will not treat a measles infection but may be prescribed to treat secondary bacterial infections that can occur as complications.

A measles vaccine, usually combined with mumps and rubella (MMR) became available in 1988 and is routinely offered to children at 15 months of age, with a booster given between six and 21 months later. It should not be given to children under 1 year old.

Seek help if your baby contracts measles before 6 months of age; if a cough lasts longer than four days and does not respond to home treatment; if your child seems no better three days after the rash has come out or gets worse after a period of recovery; if your child develops severe earache or conjunctivitis, becomes excessively drowsy, sleepy and difficult to wake and fears bright lights. These signs may signify the development of complications.

MOODINESS

Some children appear to be particularly susceptible to mood swings. They alternate between being enthusiastic and energetic to whingy and lethargic. Children who skip meals often tend to be moody and cranky. Low blood sugar levels may be to blame, particularly if mood swings usually occur in the mid-morning and mid- to late afternoon and are accompanied by feelings of weakness, faintness, irritability, hunger and nausea.

Diet and Nutritional Therapy

Regular meals are the key to keeping blood sugar levels, and moods, stable. Although sweet sugar-laden snacks such as biscuits and cakes send blood sugar levels soaring, the energy lift is only short lived. Complex carbohydrates such as bread, potatoes and pasta provide a slow but steady stream of sugar for longer-lasting benefits.

Mood swings are often a sign that certain nutrients are in short supply. A lack of vitamin B_1 and B_6 are associated with neurotic symptoms. Low amounts of the mineral magnesium, sometimes a problem in children who drink lots of milk, are linked with behavioural problems. A mood-stabilizing diet should emphasize foods rich in these nutrients.

Flower Remedies

* Chamomile (Flower Essence Society) – for those who are moody, easily upset and irritable, unable to release emotional tension, which often leads to insomnia.
* Peach-Flowered Tea-Tree (Australian Bush Essences) – for moodiness and feelings of boredom.
* Scleranthus (Bach Flower Remedies/Healing Herbs) – for mood swings, lack of concentration and restlessness.

Herbal Remedy

* Happy Child Formula (*see page 33*): 10 drops in 6 fl oz/180 ml water 3 times a day to help stabilize moods.

Professional Therapy

Homoeopathy

Professional prescribing can often help to assuage mood swings.

Doctor's Prescription

Moodiness may be related to personal worries about school or friends, so gentle enquiries about these may be helpful.
See also **Behavioural Problems**

MOUTH ULCERS

Minute white, grey or yellow spots that occur singly or in clusters in the mouth. They are often inflamed and can be painful.

There are many possible causes of mouth ulcers. They may result from biting or scratching the inside of the mouth. Food allergies or intolerances, digestive disorders, nutritional deficiencies, a viral infection or stress can also trigger mouth ulcers.

Naturopathy

The basic naturopathic diet often clears mouth ulcers. Give plenty of fresh fruits and vegetables, apple or grape juice diluted 50:50 with mineral water. Remove all processed foods from the diet.

Common triggers for mouth ulcers are chocolate and food preservatives, particularly benzoates which include E numbers 210 to 219, commonly found in fizzy drinks. Benzoates also occur naturally in tomatoes, so avoid tomato ketchup, baked beans and so forth.

Mouth ulcers can be a sign of nutritional deficiencies and allergies. They often occur when B vitamins are in short supply, but can also signify a lack of iron. To ensure a good supply of these nutrients, include plenty of wholegrain cereals and bread in your child's diet.

A daily supplement containing all the B complex vitamins and key minerals may help to clear mouth ulcers.

Homoeopathy

* Merc sol is the number one remedy for mouth ulcers. Children who need this remedy will be incredibly sensitive to heat and cold. They will often have smelly breath, be prone to swollen glands and colds and may sweat profusely. They may be extremely thirsty and salivate excessively, especially at night. Symptoms will be worse in bed at night. Give the 6C potency every 2 hours on the first day, followed by 3 times daily for 2–3 days. Stop as soon as there is some improvement.

* Alternatively, try Arsenicum album for painful ulcers on the edge of the tongue.

* Nat mur and Nit ac are also good for painful ulcers.

Other Helpful Remedies

Herbal Remedies

* Myrrh has mild antibiotic properties and makes a useful mouth wash. Add 10 drops of Myrrh tincture to 1 cup (240 ml) of warm, previously boiled water and use every morning and evening until the ulcers disappear.

* Peppermint tisane sipped regularly can help to prevent and heal mouth ulcers.

Doctor's Prescription

Antiseptic mouth rinses can be used on a short-term basis. Soluble hydrocortisone pellets or oral pastes may be prescribed.

MUMPS

A highly infectious virus which causes the parotid (salivary) glands to swell and become tender, giving rise to the characteristic hamster-cheeked appearance. Mumps is most commonly contracted between the ages of 3 and 10.

In young children the infection is often mild; many have no symptoms or are only slightly unwell. There are advantages to having this disease early in childhood, because if contracted after puberty it may have serious complications. In teenage and adult males, mumps can cause painful inflammation of one or both testes.

Incubation period: 14 to 21 days.

Infectious period: from a few days before becoming unwell until the swelling goes down, around 10 days in all.

Typical Symptoms

Discomfort and swelling in the parotid glands situated below and in front of the ears. Pain and difficulty swallowing. A feeling of sickness, headache and a temperature, which should fall after two or three days. The swelling usually subsides within a week to 10 days.

Follow the general guidelines for **Childhood Diseases**; *see also* **Infections**.

Homoeopathy

The following remedies can help to ease the discomfort of mumps and speed recovery:

> * Aconite – at the onset of symptoms of thirst, painful

throat and fever. Give 1 dose of the 6C potency every 2 or 3 hours for the first couple of days.

* Belladonna – for fever, sore throat, hot head and glassy eyes. Give a dose of the 30C potency once a day for up to 3 days or until symptoms have passed.
* Merc sol – for swelling of glands under the jaw, stitching pains to the ear on swallowing, increased saliva and bad breath. Patient will be feverish and thirsty. Give a dose of the 30C potency once a day for up to 3 days or until symptoms have passed.
* Pulsatilla – for swelling of glands under the lower jaw or testes. The sufferer will have a bad taste in the mouth and no sense of thirst, feel miserable and weepy, wanting attention. Give a dose of the 30C potency once a day for up to 3 days or until symptoms have passed.

Aromatherapy

* For children up to 5 years old: apply Tea Tree essential oil in a base of Almond Oil to the sore area, back of the neck and abdomen. Use 3 times a day for 10 days.
* For children over 5 years old: use a combination of Niaouli, Lemon and Tea Tree in a base of Almond oil; apply as above.

These essences can be added to a bowl of hot water for a steam inhalation that is decongestant and assists the body in fighting the infection. They can also be sprayed in the air with a plant spray.

Other Helpful Remedies

Naturopathy

Wrap a hot water bottle in a towel and let your child lie on it to soothe the painful swellings. For a younger baby, hold a heated towel against the face and repeat if this seems to be helping.

Diet and Nutritional Therapy

Avoid acid juices such as lemon, orange or grapefruit as these will hurt the salivary glands. Good alternatives are apple, grape and carrot.

Herbal Remedies

* Balm, Poke Root and Yarrow have a cleansing effect on the glandular system. Use singly (an infusion for Yarrow and Balm, a decoction for Poke Root) or combine all three together, sweeten with honey and give as sips 3 times a day.

Professional Therapy

Homoeopathy

While homoeopaths generally feel it is better for a child to get mumps early in childhood and establish a natural immunity for life, in some instances they can give Parotidinum 30C as a protective measure during an epidemic.

Doctor's Prescription

A paracetamol solution is generally recommended, although a child in much pain might be given painkillers.

A vaccination for mumps, usually combined with measles and

rubella vaccines (MMR) became available in 1988 and is routinely recommended at 15 months of age. It should not be given to a child under 1 year old.

Seek help if your baby or child has difficulty hearing you, becomes drowsy, unusually sensitive to light and/or develops a stiff neck.

N

NAPPY RASH

Nappy rash has several causes but most frequently results from prolonged contact with damp or soiled nappies. Irritant chemicals can form when urine and stools interact and burn the skin. Nappy rash may also occur when baby has a general infection. Residues of soap and detergents (especially non-biological washing powders) used to wash terry nappies can also irritate skin in this area. Nappy rash can also be a symptom of thrush, especially if it appears spotty, is persistent and spreads above the navel (*see* **Thrush**).

Typical Symptoms

Skin around the nappy area is sore, red and possibly spotty. May be accompanied by itching or stinging. If left untreated, painful sores may develop.

Practical Advice

Keep the skin as dry as possible by changing nappies as soon as they are wet or soiled.

Wash and rinse your baby with clean water (no soap or scented wipes), paying special attention to all the creases, wiping from front to back in girls. Pat dry with a soft towel unless the area is sore, in which case use a hairdryer on a very gentle heat.

Let baby go without a nappy for frequent periods each day. Place him on several thicknesses of towel with a plastic sheet or changing mat underneath to soak up any urine.

Try changing your brand of nappy for a more absorbent variety. Cloth nappies may be softer on the skin than disposable ones, and therefore useful during a bout of nappy rash.

Diet and Nutritional Therapy

Nappy rash is often a sign of acidic urine and digestive disturbances. Fruit juices will make the urine acidic. Give baby only plenty of plain water to drink until the rash completely clears.

* If you are breastfeeding avoid eating spicy foods, red meat, alcohol, coffee and strong tea. Avoid citrus fruits such as grapefruit and lemon as the acidity can pass from mother to baby. Drink plenty of mineral water and herbal tisanes.

* If baby is already weaned, give simple purées which are easy to digest.

* Nappy rash often clears when the diet is supplemented with essential fatty acids and vitamins A and E. These nutrients play a role in keeping the skin healthy and resilient. Try giving the contents of 2 cod liver oil capsules in a little milk or, alternatively, rub this oil into the affected area each day until the rash clears.

Other Helpful Remedies

Herbal Remedies

* Apply Calendula (marigold) cream to the area each time you change a nappy.
* Powdered Cornflower or Arrowroot make good substitutes for ordinary talcum powder, as they are soothing and will not dry the skin.

Aromatherapy

* Chamomile and Lavender are helpful for soothing and healing the skin. When washing baby's bottom add 1 drop of each essence to a bowl of warm water. Dip cotton wool in this solution, use clean cotton wool for each wipe.
* After the last nappy change before bedtime, gently apply an aromatherapy oil made with Chamomile and Lavender in a base of Jojoba oil.

Homoeopathy

* Sulphur – for a red, dry and hot rash.
* Chamomilla – when nappy rash is accompanied by green-yellow diarrhoea in angry and irritable babies.
* If breastfeeding, mother can take this remedy instead.

Give 1 dose of the 6C potency 4 times daily for up to 3 days.

Doctor's Prescription

Barrier creams and emollients along with anti-fungal agents for treating thrush may be recommended. In severe cases, corticosteroid drugs or creams may be prescribed to suppress the inflammation.

Seek help if the nappy rash fails to clear quickly, recurs frequently or raw patches develop.

NAUSEA *See* **Sickness and Nausea**

NIGHTMARES AND NIGHT TERRORS

Nightmares are vivid and upsetting dreams which often bring on feelings of anxiety and fear. No one knows for sure whether or not babies have genuine nightmares, however we do know babies dream and those who awake crying for no apparent reason may well be having bad ones. Nightmares begin to be more common around the age of 4. Research suggests that nightmares reach a peak in children aged 8 and 10 years old.

Night terrors are very different to nightmares. A child with a night terror will be screaming and sitting up in bed with eyes wide open, pupils dilated, very frightened and agitated.

Even though awake, a child suffering from a night terror will not recognize his parents and will be disorientated.

Night terrors often occur within the first 3 hours of falling asleep; it may be possible to predict when they are likely to occur. While episodes last an average of 2 minutes, they may go on for up to 20. Night terrors can be averted if you awaken a child who is sweating, tossing and turning.

Practical Advice

Children are very impressionable: alarming images on television, even in the form of cartoons, may contribute to nightmares and night terrors. As a precautionary measure it may be a good idea to vet or even limit your child's television viewing, especially in the evening.

Give gentle reassurance to a child awaking from a nightmare. It helps a child just to know you are close and he is quite safe. Try talking about a comforting and happy subject as this diverts the mind away from the nightmare. Cuddle a child with a night terror until he settles down and goes back to sleep.

Flower Remedies

* Aspen (Bach Flower Remedies/Healing Herbs) – for those who wake in fear and panic, scared to go back to sleep.
* Green Spider Orchid (Australian Bush Flower Essences) for nightmares and phobias. Brings release from terror.
* Rock Rose (Bach Flower Remedies/ Healing Herbs) – for extreme terror and panic nearing hysteria.
* St John's Wort (Deva Flower Elixirs) – for children prone to restless dreams, nightmares, nocturnal fears, night terrors and fear of death.

Give 2 drops at bedtime and again if your child wakes during the night.

Homoeopathy

* Phosphorus – for those who hate to be alone, especially in the dark at night when their vivid imaginations go to work. They are scared of thunderstorms, sensitive, highly strung and easily startled. Respond well to massage, touch and affection.
* Stramonium – for babies who are terrified of the dark and wake up with frightful nightmares, recognizing no one. They have a strange fear of water and glittering surfaces such as mirrors. Prone to tantrums as soon as they are mobile.

Give 1 dose of the 30c potency, watch for improvement and repeat if there is some relief for up to 3 doses.

Other Helpful Remedies

Herbal Remedy

* Give Chamomile tisane to sip just before bedtime.

Aromatherapy

Place a tissue sprinkled with Chamomile and Orange essential oils under your child's pillow. You could also use these essences in a vaporizer.

NOSEBLEEDS

Nosebleeds are very common in children and are not usually a cause for concern. They can result from a knock which damages the delicate blood vessels inside the nose. Nosebleeds may accompany a heavy cold or nasal infection.

Practical Advice

Your child should sit up and, with the head slightly bent forward, pinch the bridge of the nose firmly between the thumb and forefinger. Keep the pressure up until the bleeding stops.

Lying down is not recommended as it forces the blood down the throat.

Try pressing the acupressure point between the tip of the nose and lip for 30 to 60 seconds.

Diet and Nutritional Therapy

Frequent nosebleeds can signify a shortage of vitamin C and bioflavonoids. The bioflavonoids occur naturally with vitamin C and play an important role in keeping the tiny blood capillaries lining the nose healthy. Give 500 mg (250 mg for under-threes) of vitamin C with bioflavonoids daily for 2 weeks.

Homoeopathy

* Aconite – for nosebleeds triggered by a shock or fright.
* Arnica – for nosebleeds that occur after an injury or trauma to the nose, or following a coughing fit.
* Ferrum phos – for bright red nosebleeds in children.
* Phosphorus – for frequent nosebleeds that occur for no apparent reason.

Give 1 dose of the 6c or 30c potency immediately.

Other Helpful Remedies

Herbal Remedy

* Witch hazel is an astringent that helps to stop bleeding. Add 15 drops to 1 cup (240 ml) of cooled boiled water. Saturate a piece of cotton wool in this solution and hold under the nose.

Doctor's Prescription

Cautery to 'Little's Avea', an area rich in small blood vessels just inside the nose, may be necessary for repetitive bleeds.

P

PHOBIAS

An irrational and disabling fear of specific things such as spiders, snakes and ghosts, or situations like being in the dark and thunder storms. Older children may be particularly fearful of death, crowds, strangers and loud noises.

Phobias can be the result of previous unpleasant experiences. They can also be learned or acquired from parents and siblings.

Phobias are difficult to treat on your own, and natural remedies can only help to soothe an agitated child. If phobias seriously impair your child's enjoyment of life it is important to seek professional help.

Typical Symptoms

Extreme anxiety and fear accompanied with rapid breathing, sweating, panic and general depression. Anxiety about certain things may manifest as nightmares, sleep-walking and teeth grinding.

Diet and Nutritional Therapy

Research suggests that people who suffer from phobias experience symptoms similar to those with low blood sugar.

Keeping blood sugar levels stable with small, frequent meals may help to prevent attacks. Stabilizing foods are the complex carbohydrates (potatoes, wholegrain breads and cereals, rice and pasta). Sweet, sugary foods should be avoided.

Flower Remedies

* Mimulus (Bach Flower Remedies/Healing Herbs) – for fears of specific or known origin often undisclosed due to shyness.
* Rock Rose (Bach Flower Remedies/Healing Herbs) – for extreme terror and panic nearing hysteria.
* An emergency composite for treating shock and trauma such as Rescue Remedy (Bach Flower Remedies) or Five Flower Remedy (Healing Herbs) is good to give in anticipation of fearfulness (i.e. before bedtime) as well as straight after an alarming event.

Give 2 drops under the tongue or in water every hour until the fear subsides.

Other Helpful Remedies

Aromatherapy and Massage

* The aroma of Lavender provides quick relief from anxiety

and fearfulness. Sprinkle a few drops on a handkerchief and tuck this into your child's pocket or under his pillow so it is always at hand. Refresh the aroma on a regular basis.

* A soothing back massage will help to reassure and calm a panicky child. Add a few drops of Lavender to your chosen carrier oil.

Professional Therapy

Homoeopathy

A professional homoeopath can prescribe an appropriate remedy for children of a fearful disposition.

Compare **Anxiety, Depression, Nightmares and Night Terrors**

PSORIASIS

A skin condition characterized by thick, red patches covered with a distinctive silvery sheen, usually present on bony areas of the body such as the shins, elbows or scalp.

Psoriasis is caused by the over-production of skin cells which appears to be an inherited (genetic) tendency, but is also aggravated by stress or trauma. It is a fairly uncommon condition in children. An estimated 1 per cent of the population may develop psoriasis at some time in their lives.

Naturopathy

Naturopaths recommend the basic naturopathic diet (*see page 48*), exposing skin to plenty of natural sunlight and bathing in sea water. At home the benefits of sea bathing can be recreated by tossing a handful of sea salt into the bath.

The minerals from the Dead Sea are renowned for being helpful to psoriasis sufferers due to the high proportion of magnesium and bromine, which have relaxing properties. Dead Sea salts can be bought from most good healthfood stores.

An oatmeal bath helps to soothe irritated skin. Put 5 tablespoons of fine oatmeal in a cheesecloth or muslin bag. Place in a hot bath and soak for 15 minutes.

Essential fatty acids found in oily fish such as salmon, mackerel and sardines may be beneficial. Daily supplements of cod liver oil are a useful alternative for children who are not keen on fish.

Some psoriasis sufferers benefit from taking Evening Primrose Oil: 1 × 500-mg capsule a day for 2 to 3 months.

Herbal Remedies

Many cases of psoriasis respond to herbal remedies prescribed to suit the individual by a professional herbalist. Safe home remedies to try are Yarrow and Burdock root:

* Make an infusion of Yarrow by adding 1 oz/30 g to 1 pint/600 ml of water, then add this to the bath water twice a week to help clear impurities from the skin. The infusion may also be sipped, preferably a little each day to bring the best results. Yarrow herb can be placed in a muslin bag which, when damp, can be used as a compress and to scrub patches of psoriasis.

* Burdock root is an excellent remedy for dry, scaly skin. Make a decoction by adding 1 teaspoon of root to 1 pint/600 ml of water, simmer for 15 minutes, strain and give as a drink 3 times a day.

* An ointment containing Burdock will also help to relieve the irritation and scaliness. Ask a herbalist to make a special preparation for you.

* Macerated Calendula oil can help to soothe psoriasis.

* You can also add 1 cup of Chickweed tea to the bath.

* Immune Balance Formula (*see page 32*): 10 drops in 6 fl oz/180 ml water 2 times a day whenever psoriasis flares up.

Other Helpful Remedies

Aromatherapy

* Gently massage the affected areas with Lavender in a carrier of Almond, Avocado or Rosehip oil.
* For children over 7 years old: Use a blend of equal proportions of Lavender and Bergamot (4–6 drops of each in 30 ml of carrier oil).

Relaxation

Stress can aggravate psoriasis. A full body massage will help to induce feelings of relaxation. Practising some kind of relaxation therapy on a regular basis is also helpful for controlling anxiety and tension.

Professional Therapies

Homoeopathy

Remedies will be tailored to the individual and take into account all other symptoms.

Chinese Medicine

This can be effective at treating various skin diseases including psoriasis. Consult a qualified practitioner.

Doctor's Prescription

As with eczema, this is a chronic condition and as such there is no absolute cure, although measures can be taken to minimize and dampen down flare-ups.

Medical treatment consists of creams, lotions and shampoos containing coal tar extract, salicylic acid, dithranol and newer vitamin D derivatives. These help to decrease skin cell turnover.

Severe psoriasis is sometimes treated with a combination of psoralins and UV light. An outbreak may follow a viral infection, such as a fever.

Compare **Eczema**

R

RASHES

There are various different kinds of rashes. Some are caused by heat while others may be the symptom of an allergic reaction or eczema. Rashes may also accompany certain infectious diseases. Heat rashes will be considered here, as the others are dealt with elsewhere in the book (*see* **Eczema**, **Childhood Diseases**, **Hives**)

Typical Symptoms

Tiny red blotches usually appearing in areas of concentrated heat: the nappy area, under the arms, in the neck folds, tummy and so forth.

There is a tendency to think that newborn babies need to be wrapped up in layer upon layer of baby clothes and shawls. As babies cannot remove any unwanted layers they can become overheated; in extreme cases this may be dangerous.

As a general rule baby will only need a cotton vest, babygrow and cardigan for indoors. For outdoors the number of layers added will depend on the temperature.

You can easily check if baby is too warm by slipping two fingers inside his vest.

Other Helpful Remedies

Aromatherapy

Add Lavender and Chamomile to the bath. These essential oils are suitable for newborn babies.

Chinese Medicine

Traditionally this involves applying a paste of Mung Bean powder mixed with water to the skin.

Herbal Remedies

* Aloe Vera gel will cool and soothe a heat rash.
* Bathe the area with Chickweed tea, or a cupful to the bath.

See also **Nappy Rash**

RINGWORM

A fungal infection of the skin characterized by red, scaly circular patches with clear centres. The name comes from this 'ring' shape and is not caused by a worm at all. If ringworm forms on the scalp it can cause temporary hair loss. It may also affect the nails.

Ringworm is infectious and may be caught from domestic and farm animals as well as other people.

Practical Advice

Scrupulous hygiene is essential in clearing this problem, as are external healing treatments. If the condition persists you will need to seek professional help.

Aromatherapy

* For children over 2 years old: apply 1 drop of neat Tea Tree oil over the affected area 3 times a day until it clears. This should take no more than 10 days.
* Make an aromatherapy oil containing equal proportions of Lavender and Tea Tree in 30 ml of Almond oil and rub over the area daily.

Herbal Remedies

* Bathe with a tincture of Myrrh and rub Garlic oil into the affected areas.
* Echinacea will help to strengthen the immune system in its attempts to clear the fungal infection. Add up to 15 drops of Echinacea tincture to 1 cup (240 ml) of cooled boiled water and give as sips 3 times a day.

Other Helpful Remedies

Homoeopathy

* Psor – ringworm all over the body.
* Sepia – for isolated spots on the upper part of the body only.

Give 1 dose of the 30C potency daily for 3 days. It may be a good idea to seek professional advice from a homoeopath.

Doctor's Prescription

Anti-fungal creams such as Canasten (clotrimazole) with or without a mild steroid to reduce inflammation are likely to be prescribed.
Compare **Eczema**, **Psoriasis**

RUBELLA (GERMAN MEASLES)

A mild infection in children which is usually no worse than a cold and lasts for about 3 to 5 days. Rubella most commonly occurs between the ages of 6 and 12. An attack confers life-long immunity. It is important to keep a child with Rubella away from any woman who is pregnant or trying for a child. If Rubella is contracted during the first 4 months of pregnancy there is a risk of damage to the unborn baby.

Incubation period: 14 to 21 days.

Infectious period: 1 week before and at least 4 days after the rash first appears.

Typical Symptoms

Begins like a mild cold. A faint pink rash of tiny flat spots appears behind the ears and spreads down the body. Glands in the neck may be swollen. Sometimes accompanied by a sore throat and watery eyes. A baby may be grizzly for few days before the rash comes out and could have a fever without other symptoms. A young child is unlikely to feel particularly unwell.

Follow the general guidelines for **Childhood Diseases**; *see also* **Infections**.

Homoeopathy

* Euphrasia – for a rash with cold symptoms, cough, eye inflammation. Fever not usually very high; patient does not necessarily feel very ill.
* Pulsatilla – for rash accompanied by yellow mucus, sore inflamed eyes and cough with characteristic weepiness and lack of thirst.

Give the 6C potency every hour for up to 6 doses. Repeat if necessary. You can also give the Recipe for Spotty Illnesses (see page 101–2).

Aromatherapy

* For babies and children over 6 months: Combine 10 drops of Lavender, 10 drops of Chamomile and 4 drops of Tea Tree in 30 ml of Almond oil.
* Add 4 drops of this blend to 1 pint/600 ml warm water and use to sponge down the body once a day.
* Add the appropriate number of drops (*see page 6*) to a bedtime bath.
* Use this blend in a vaporizer to cleanse the air.

Other Helpful Remedies

Herbal Remedy

* Yarrow infusion can help to clear the symptoms. Pour 1 cup/240 ml of boiling water over 1 teaspoon of the dried herb, infuse for 10 minutes, strain and sweeten with honey to taste. Give hot as sips 3 times a day.

Professional Therapy

Homoeopathy

It is generally considered better to have German Measles during childhood, but Rubella 30 can be given as a protective measure during an epidemic.

Doctor's Prescription

Children should stay at home while they have a rash and for three days after the spots have disappeared. If there is a temperature they should stay in bed. Rubella is a mild illness and does not usually need treatment.

A Rubella vaccine, given in combination with Measles and Mumps (MMR) is routinely offered to infants at around 15 months old. It is not recommended for children under 1 year old.

Seek help if there is a high fever, marked drowsiness and your baby cries persistently. Encephalitis is a rare complication which may occur in 1 in 6,000 cases.

S

SHOCK

A sudden shock has a shattering effect on children as well as adults. The mind is temporarily unable to concentrate or focus on anything and emotions are heightened. Shock has a 'freezing' effect on the tissues and all the muscles, which in turn makes breathing rapid and shallow.

Some degree of shock can occur after any injury or illness, especially if it involves a loss of blood or other bodily fluids. It can also occur during and infection or allergic reaction.

Children recover from shock in their own time, though it leave its imprint on the mind and body unless steps are taken to undo the damage. The birth process may be a shocking experience for many babies. Natural remedies can help babies who are obviously distressed and cry a great deal after birth.

Typical Symptoms

General weakness, cold, clammy, pale skin, a rapid, weak pulse, shallow, irregular breathing, reduced alertness and an inability to focus attention. There may also be a feeling of nausea.

Homoeopathy

* Aconite – for shock with extreme fear and panic; for nightmares following shock. Arnica is also the number one remedy for shock resulting from an accident or physical injury.

Give the 30C dose immediately and follow with another 1 to 2 doses if needed.

Flower Remedies

* Arnica (Deva Flower Elixirs) – to be taken after any physical, mental or emotional trauma.
* Emergency Essence (Jan de Vries) – a blend of essences of Chamomile, Lavender, Red Clover, Purple Coneflower, Self-Heal and Yarrow. Has a gentle calming and re-balancing action.
* First Aid Remedy (Findhorn Flower Essences) – a composite of flower remedies which can help to relieve the after-effects of shock.
* Star of Bethlehem (Bach Flower Remedies/Healing Herbs) – for all forms of shock, including the shock of birth.

Other Helpful Remedies

Herbal Remedy

* Sweet Peppermint tea is a good remedy for counteracting shock.

Chinese Medicine

* Liquorice tincture in warm (previously boiled) water.

Massage

Lightly touching a hand or foot can help to calm an agitated child. As the shock subsides you can try working the solar plexus reflex area (*see Figure 2, page 53*).

Professional Therapy

Osteopathy

An osteopath may actually feel the presence of shock in the body. Consult a qualified practitioner.

SICKNESS AND NAUSEA

Feeling and or being sick is usually a sign of having eaten something which the body cannot tolerate; spontaneous rejection serves as form of protection. It is most commonly a symptom of food poisoning and is triggered by toxins produced by undesirable bacteria. Sickness and nausea may also accompany ear infections and infectious illnesses in general.

The symptoms can be produced by the motion of travelling by car, train, boat or aeroplane as well as more vigorous movements such as fun-fair rides *see* **Travel Sickness**. Vomiting can also be associated with worms and with painful injuries with an element of shock.

Emotional upsets such as fear, shock and anxiety can also bring on nausea and vomiting – pre-exam nerves being the classic example.

Typical Symptoms

Feeling queasy, faint, dizzy and shaky, sometimes leading to regurgitation of stomach contents.

Young babies frequently posset (throw up) small amounts of their feed and this is generally considered normal. Babies up to 1 year old can have a mild stomach bug with sickness and diarrhoea without any serious side-effects.

If a baby vomits frequently and has a fever, food poisoning is the most likely cause.

A baby who is constantly being sick may be allergic to a particular food, possibly cow's milk. Very rarely, babies suffer from projectile vomiting when the stomach contents are hurled violently across the room, a condition that requires medical treatment.

The following treatments will ease feelings of nausea and provide relief after an attack of vomiting. If your baby or child has an episode of vomiting lasting more than 1 or 2 hours you should consult your doctor. Sickness can be a sign of a serious illness such as meningitis or kidney infection. Always act quickly with infants as they can become dehydrated very quickly.

Practical Advice

Vomiting can be frightening for a baby so do hold him during the sickness. Once it is over give reassuring cuddles.

Encourage a baby or young child to take a little water to rinse out his mouth. Do not let him have too much until you are sure it is staying down.

Being sick can be exhausting, so encourage your baby or small child to lie down and rest for at least half a day afterwards.

Diet and Nutritional Therapy

* It is best to abstain from food altogether until the nausea and sickness subsides. Give plenty of fluids to prevent dehydration (around 2–3 pints a day if possible).
* Add 1 teaspoon of salt and 2 dessertspoons of sugar to 2 pints/1 litre of boiled water; add 1 pint (600 ml) of orange or lemon juice. Give a glass of this mixture every hour after a bout of vomiting.
* If you are breastfeeding you can carry on nursing your baby even if some of the feed comes up again. As well as providing him nourishment, this will also be a source of comfort.
* When reintroducing solids, choose bland, non-fatty foods such as yoghurt, toast and honey.
* Nausea and vomiting sometimes signify a lack of vitamin B_6. Breastfed babies are less likely to be sick than those given formula. However breastmilk is not particularly rich in vitamin B, so sicky babies may benefit if mother takes 25 mg of vitamin B_6 after each meal for a short while.

Homoeopathy

* Arsenicum is the number one remedy for food poisoning. The child who needs this remedy will bring back everything he eats immediately until nothing is left in the stomach. He will be fearful of being sick, feel chilly and headachy, and be unable to bear the sight, smell or thought of food. Feelings of nausea will be intense.
* Ipecac is the chosen remedy for persistent nausea that is unrelieved by vomiting. Other signs include a clean tongue, dry cough and gagging.

* Nux vom – for nausea with or without vomiting which occurs after eating rich or unusual foods.

Other Helpful Remedies

Herbal Remedies

* Ginger is an effective remedy for nausea. Make a weak Ginger tea by soaking 1 teaspoon of Ginger root in 1 cup (240 ml) of boiled water, strain, add honey to taste. Alternatively, give crystallized ginger to suck.
* Peppermint helps to relieve nausea and settle the stomach after being sick. Give sips of Peppermint infusion, or Peppermint tablets to suck.
* Infusions or tinctures of Meadowsweet and/or Lemon Balm can also help to soothe and settle the stomach.

Massage

Work the Pericardium 6 acupressure point (as for **Travel Sickness**; *see Figure 1, page 13*). A child can also be taught how to find and massage this point as a self-help measure.

Aromatherapy

For children over 1 year old: use Peppermint only. Sprinkle onto a tissue for your child to inhale and add to a base of Almond oil for massaging the stomach.

For children over 5 years old: you can also use Sandalwood.

For children over 7 years old: you can also use Melissa and Basil. Any of these four essential oils can be used singly or in a blend.

Doctor's Prescription

This will depend on the cause of the vomiting. Doctors generally recommend avoiding food until the sickness is over and giving Dioralyte (rehydration mix) after a bout of sickness to safeguard against dehydration.

Seek help if your baby or child vomits incessantly, as this is always a serious symptom. It may indicate an emergency such as an obstruction. Make sure your child lies on his side so he cannot inhale the vomit.

If there is any sign of dehydration – a dry mouth and lips, dark concentrated urine or no urine for longer than 6 hours, sunken eyes, abnormal drowsiness or lethargy; if your baby or child vomits after a fall on the head; if your baby is vomiting a fair amount without otherwise seeming ill and is not gaining any weight, do contact your doctor.

SINUSITIS

Infection or inflammation of the sinus cavities, often accompanied by excessive catarrh. Acute sinusitis may be accompanied by a fever and severe headache. This condition is often aggravated by colds, hay fever, emotional upset or damp weather.

Typical Symptoms

Pain at the root of the nose and above or below the eyes. A feeling of stuffiness in the head.

Follow recommendations for treating **Colds**.

Other Helpful Remedies

Naturopathy

* Naturopaths recommend avoiding milk and all dairy products to clear excessive catarrh.
* Elderflower tisane, sipped when hot, will encourage catarrh flow and help to relieve sinusitis.
* Garlic has antibiotic properties and helps to prevent and clear infection. Give 2 capsules at bedtime.

Homoeopathy

* Kali bich – for pressure or bunged-up sensation at the root of the nose. Thick, stringy, yellow discharge. Painful headache, especially over the eyebrows.

Give 1 dose of the 30C potency once a day for 3 days.

Biochemic Tissue Salts

* Combination Q: 2 tablets 3 times daily.

Aromatherapy

* For children over 5 years old: give a steam inhalation by adding 2 drops of Eucalyptus and 2 drops of Thyme essential oils to a bowl of hot water. Cover the head with a towel and encourage deep breaths of the vapours. Always supervise steam inhalation.
* Gently massage with these essences (4 drops of each in 30 ml of carrier oil) into the forehead and down each side of the nose. Rub a little oil into the chest to ease breathing at night.

See also **Colds, Hay Fever, Infections**

SLEEPING PROBLEMS

Most parents experience problems with getting their baby or child to sleep soundly through the night at some time or another.

Sleeping problems are so common that many books have been written on this subject and practical advice on ways to get your child to sleep abounds.

In young babies, sleeping problems at night are invariably to be expected. While some fall into good sleeping patterns early on, others take much longer to be persuaded to sleep during the night hours.

A breastfed baby will tend to wake more frequently because mother's milk is easily assimilated and after about 3 or 4 hours baby will be ready for more. Breastfed babies can feed in the night without really waking up and are easily put back to bed again.

Some babies are difficult to put to sleep and may wake frequently at night for no apparent reason – a problem which can often be relieved with the appropriate homoeopathic remedy (*see below*).

Sleep problems in children can occur for a number of possible reasons. Always check:

* Is your child too hot or too cold?
* Hungry?
* Uncomfortable due to a blocked nose, cough, eczema, stomach ache etc.?
* Full of pent-up energy due to lack of exercise?
* Anxious due to upheavals such as moving house, changing school?
* Apprehensive about being alone in the dark due to night fears and phobias?

Falling asleep is a skill that needs to be cultivated. If babies or children go to bed when they are over-excited they will find it difficult to drift off. About an hour before bedtime, try to create an environment that is as conducive to relaxation and sleep. Reading books, singing nursery rhymes and listening to soothing music can all help to send babies and children off to sleep.

There are also natural remedies for encouraging relaxation at the end of the day and easing any physical or emotional problems which can interfere with a sound night's sleep.

Aromatherapy and Massage

After a bath or just before bedtime, try to establish a routine of giving your child a gentle massage with a soothing aromatherapy oil.

Babies are much easier to massage after a bath than are young children, who are much more bouncy at this time. It may be best to wait until your child has settled down for a bedtime read before giving him a gentle back rub or hand and foot massage.

Most children, like grown-ups, can be sent off to sleep when stroked on a particular spot such as the forehead. You can also concentrate on massaging the 'insomnia' acupressure point (Heart 7: *see Figure 1, page 13*).

* For young babies: use Chamomile in a base of Almond oil.
* For babies over 1 year old: you can also use Geranium.
* For children over 6 years old: combine Chamomile and Geranium together.

Add these essences to a warm bath to help your child to unwind and to induce feelings of calmness. You can also use them in a vaporizer in the bedroom and/or place a few drops on a tissue and tuck it under your child's pillow.

Herbal Remedies

Many herbs are effective sedatives and will encourage wakeful infants to drift off to sleep. Valerian is particularly potent and has been used as a tranquillizer for over 1,000 years – as such it should only be prescribed by a professional herbalist. If your child always has difficulty getting to sleep consult a professional herbalist, who can make up an appropriate blend.

* For occasional bouts of sleeplessness, infusions of Passionflower, Chamomile, Orange Blossom, Balm and Lime flowers can do the trick. Try combining 2 or 3 of these herbs together. Sweeten with honey and give by the teaspoon for babies and as sips from a small teacup for children over 3 years old.

* Drops of Lemon Balm (Melissa) or Passionflower (*Passiflora*) tincture can also be added to warm milk or fruit juice.

* A sleep-inducing bath can be created by adding an infusion of Hops to the water. Either infuse 1 oz/30 g of Hops in boiling water for 10 minutes or tie them up in a muslin bag and hang from the hot tap so water pours through the Hops as it runs into the bath.

Other Helpful Remedies

Diet and Nutritional Therapy

* A milky drink before bedtime has long been recognized as encouraging sleepiness. Milk is a rich source of an amino acid called tryptophan which the body converts into serotonin, a brain chemical involved with regulating sleep patterns and feelings of tranquillity. Other good sources of tryptophan are bananas, avocados, figs and pineapple.

* The mineral zinc may also be involved in healthy sleep patterns. Research suggests that babies who wake one or more times a night between midnight and 7 a.m. sleep more soundly when given 12 mg of

elemental zinc.
* Magnesium and calcium, sometimes refereed to as nature's tranquillizers, are also involved in the ability to sleep soundly.

Homoeopathy

There are many possible remedies for treating sleeplessness, which is invariably part of a symptom pattern and ideally should be treated by a professional homoeopath.

The following ones are often useful for easing sleep problems in babies and children.

* Borax – for babies who wake screaming from the slightest noise or for no apparent reason, as if from a nightmare. If asleep when placed in their cot they wake immediately, as they dislike downward movement.
* Calc carb – for sleeplessness caused by worry, with persistently restless thoughts and anxious dreams.
* Coffea – for children who sleep lightly, waking at every sound, unable to sleep because of excitement, ideas and plans.
* Magnesia mur – for those who are restless and anxious in bed, especially on closing eyes; may be oversensitive to noise and unable to get to sleep.
* Stramonium – for babies who are terrified of the dark and wake up with nightmares, recognizing no one.

Give 1 dose of the 30C remedy, wait to see if there is any improvement and, if so, repeat for up to 3 doses.

Relaxation

Various relaxation techniques can be beneficial when sleeplessness is linked to stress and anxiety.

Chinese Medicine

The Heart 7 acupressure point, also known as the *Shen Men* or 'Door of the Mind', is one of the basic points for treating insomnia. One study showed that sleep problems in children aged 5–6 improved when this point was stimulated (*see Figure 1, page 13*).

Reflexology

Work the solar plexus reflex area on the hands and feet (*see Figure 2, page 13*).

Flower Remedies

* Hop's Bush (Australian Living Essences) – for those who cannot sleep or relax due to frenetic energy.
* Valerian (Deva Flower Elixirs) – to overcome insomnia, stress and nervous irritation.

Professional Therapy

Osteopathy

Sleeping problems in babies can be linked to birth trauma and often respond to subtle manipulative treatment. Consult a professional osteopath.

Doctor's Prescription

The use of strong sedatives is not encouraged. If parents are desperate, a small dose of Phenergan may be recommended.

Compare **Nightmares and Night Terrors**

SORE THROAT

A sore throat usually signifies the onset of an illness such as a cold, influenza, croup or laryngitis. As the illness develops, the sore throat usually gets better. While sore throats are usually caused by viruses, they may also result from the *Streptococcus* bacteria (so-called strep throat), which sometimes develops into a more serious problem. If the sore throat does not feel better within a couple of days or a high fever develops, consult your doctor.

Sore throats are usually self-limiting and symptoms will go with rest. Meanwhile, natural remedies can help to relieve the discomfort and hasten recovery.

Typical Symptoms

A rasping, raw sensation in the throat. Glands in the neck may feel swollen and tender to touch. In babies the voice may sound hoarse or lower in tone. They may cry when eating or drinking because swallowing is painful.

Diet and Nutritional Therapy

* Offer plenty of fluids. Breastmilk is ideal, interspersed with a little freshly squeezed orange or lemon juice diluted with cooled boiled water and sweetened with honey. This may be offered by spoon if baby does not want to drink from a bottle or beaker.
* Vitamin C can help to speed recovery, so give plenty of vitamin C-rich fruits and vegetables.
* The mineral zinc will support the immune system and can help to reduce the duration of a cold. Good natural sources are fish and lean meat. Freshly made chicken and vegetable soup is a good natural remedy for a sore throat.

* Bilberries, blackberries and blackcurrants have slightly antiseptic properties and are recommended for throat infections including laryngitis and tonsillitis. Squeeze fresh fruit, dilute with a little warm (previously boiled) water, strain and add honey to taste.

* These fruits can also be made into an excellent soothing syrup for sore throats, but you will need to make it before the cold season gets underway: Mix together 4 oz (120 g) of fresh fruit and the same quantity of sugar, place in a saucepan and heat. Add 2 tablespoons of gin or vodka. Leave to macerate in a cool place for a few weeks. Strain, bottle and keep in the fridge for when it is needed.

Herbal Remedies

* Garlic can help to fight the viral and bacterial infections responsible for sore throats. Use plenty of garlic in cooking or give 3 Garlic oil tablets daily.

* Red Sage makes an effective gargle for an inflamed throat. Make an infusion and use warm, twice a day for 5 minutes each time. This may also be drunk as a soothing tea.

* Cinnamon and Ginger can help to ease the sore throats associated with colds. Warm a little fruit juice such as pineapple, grape or apple in a saucepan and sprinkle in about half a teaspoon of powdered Cinnamon or Ginger for a comforting drink.

* Elderflower Syrup (*see page 31*) can help to soothe a sore throat: 1 teaspoon 3 times a day.

Other Helpful Remedies

Homoeopathy

* Aconite – for a sudden sore throat made worse by cold wind. Signs will include a burning throat, swollen tonsils and a bitter taste in the mouth.
* Gelsemium – for pain in the neck, painful on swallowing; sufferer will feel weak and exhausted.
* Try Belladonna or Lycopodium if the pain is right-sided; Lacheris or Merc sol if the pain is left-sided.

Give 1 dose of the 6C potency 3 times a day for up 6 doses.

Aromatherapy

* For babies up to 6 months old: add Lavender or Chamomile to a base of Almond oil and gently rub into the chest and throat area.
* For babies over 6 months old: Tea Tree can be also be used.
* For children over 6 years old: Lemon and Ginger can be added to this repertoire, used alone or in simple blends of two essences of your choice.
* Make a mouthwash with 4 drops of either Lavender, Chamomile, Lemon, Ginger or Tea Tree oil in 50 ml of tepid (previously boiled) water. Pour a small amount into a glass and ask your child to take a mouthful, swishing the mixture around his mouth for 30 seconds. It also helps to gargle with the mixture before spitting it away.

Chinese Medicine

* Give Peppermint tisane to sip.

* Massage the Large Intestine 4 acupressure point (*see Figure 1, page 13*).

Biochemic Tissue Salts

* Ferr phos: 3 tablets every hour until symptoms improve.

Doctor's Prescription

Gargling with salt water is often recommended, along with paracetamol solution to ease the pain. Antibiotics may be prescribed for severe cases of strep throat.

Seek help if your baby or child is dribbling excessively, has difficulty breathing and great pain in swallowing, if very distressed and obviously not reacting to home prescribing quickly (within a day or two).

See also **Colds, Croup, Influenza, Laryngitis**

STINGS *See* **Bites and Stings**

STOMACH ACHE (ABDOMINAL PAIN)

Stomach aches and pains have many different causes: indigestion or food poisoning, food allergy/intolerance or a sign of coeliac disease, especially when there is bloating and excessive wind. Pains in the abdominal area may accompany urinary infections. Children are particularly prone to nervous stomach aches and they are often a sign of anxiety, worry and tension. Abdominal pains may also indicate a more serious condition such as appendicitis, which often begins as a mild stomach ache. If the pain lasts for more than 6 hours or is accompanied by feelings of dizziness, sweating, pallor or vomiting, consult your doctor straight away.

Naturopathy

As a preventative measure, give a simple wholefood diet with plenty of fresh vegetables and fruits, wholegrain cereals, fresh fish, poultry and natural yoghurt. Limit fatty and sugar-laden foods as much as possible.

Try applying the principles of food combining to make digestion easier. In its simplest form this involves eating protein-rich foods such as fish, meat and cheese at separate meals from carbohydrate-rich foods such as bread, cereals and potatoes. Most vegetables combine well with either of these food groups.

The Food Combining Diet by Kathryn Marsden (Thorsons) provides more detail on this way of eating.

It is best to avoid food until the stomach ache passes. Afterwards give a little grated raw carrot and apple to soothe the stomach.

Herbal Remedies

* Slippery Elm is renowned for its calming effect on the digestive system. The powdered bark (available from healthfood stores) can be stirred into a hot milky drink or warmed fruit juice. It can also be taken in tablet form after meals.

* Chamomile, Peppermint and Meadowsweet tisanes are good for the digestion and will also help to soothe stomach ache when sipped after mealtimes.

* Grated Ginger root tea sweetened with honey will also help to remove feelings of nausea.

Other Helpful Remedies

Chinese Medicine

* Ginger or Liquorice tincture in warm (previously boiled) water.

* Work the Stomach 25 acupressure point (*see Figure 1, page 13*).

Homoeopathy

The most appropriate remedy depends on what kind of sensation is being experienced (stabbing or shooting pains, dull ache, etc.), which it can be difficult for a young child to describe.

* For babies – *see* **Colic**.
* Colocynthis – stomach/abdomen feels bloated, pains are cutting, griping, violent and come in waves, with diarrhoea, nausea, vomiting. Eating, especially fruit, will aggravate the pain.
* Dioscorea – abdomen/stomach rumbles, windiness. Cramping pain around the navel. An infant arches his back and does not want to lie down, better for being upright.

Give 1 dose of the 6C potency every hour for up to 4 doses.

Biochemic Tissue Salts

* Try Mag phos or Combination E: 2 tablets every hour for up to 6 doses.

Aromatherapy and Massage

Make an aromatherapy oil and massage the stomach using gentle but firm circular strokes with the three middle fingers, working around the abdomen in a clockwise direction.

* For babies up to 6 months old: use Lavender or Dill in a base of Almond oil.
* For children over 1 year old: you can also use Peppermint and Geranium, but choose just one essence.

* For children over 6: you can also use Rosemary, combining any two of the recommended essences, such as Lavender and Peppermint or Geranium and Rosemary.

Flower Remedies

* Chamomile (Flower Essence Society) – particularly good for those who are easily upset, moody and irritable, unable to release emotional tension.

Doctor's Prescription

This will depend on the cause of the stomach ache. Urinary infections are best dealt with medically, and will be treated with antibiotics. Constipation can also cause recurrent pain, and migraine can present as abdominal pain in childhood.
See also **Coeliac Disease**, **Constipation**

SUNBURN

The delicate skin of babies and children is easily burnt by the sun's rays; exposure should be kept to a bare minimum.

Sunburn is itself very painful in the short term, and in the long term it can do lasting damage. Young skin is unable to repair all the harm caused by sunburn and it is now thought that overexposure to the sun's rays in childhood can damage the skin for life, only revealing itself years later. Early sun damage is now thought to be a major contributor to premature wrinkling and possibility even skin cancer.

Sun protection is vital for all babies and young children. The best form is protective clothing and sun hats, although a sun block cream is also recommended for the face and any other exposed areas. Always choose at least a factor 15 preparation offering protection from both UVB and UVA rays.

Sun creams need to be reapplied every 2 hours to ensure they work effectively. A waterproof or water-resistant preparation is best if your child is swimming or paddling.

Typical Symptoms

Pink or reddened skin which is painful to touch. Sunburnt skin may blister and peel after a day or two, in which case extra care must be taken to protect the underlying skin.

Herbal Remedies

* Aloe Vera is recommended for all kinds of burns due to its cooling, soothing, moisturizing and healing properties. Dab the skin with cotton wool soaked in Aloe Vera juice, or smother affected areas with Aloe Vera gel.
* Apply Hypericum (St John's Wort) oil or ointment to sunburnt skin.
* An infusion of Chamomile flowers can be used to sponge down sore, sunburnt areas.

Other Helpful Remedies

Naturopathy

Apply cool yoghurt straight from the fridge. Leave on the skin for as long as it is tolerated before wiping away.

Aromatherapy

* Add Lavender or Tea Tree to a sponge-down solution and to the bath; add to a carrier of Rosehip oil for rubbing gently into the skin.

Homoeopathy

If sunburn is accompanied by sunstroke, give the appropriate remedy (*see* **Sunstroke**).

Doctor's Prescription

If the sunburn is severe or covers a large area, fluid replacements and dressings are needed.

SUNSTROKE

Being in the sun for long periods can give rise to sunstroke. In general children are unable to tolerate the heat as well as adults. Even a few hours' outdoors on a hot summer's day may result in mild symptoms of sunstroke.

Typical Symptoms

Feeling over-heated, restless, faint, headachy, nauseous and fatigued. More severe sunstroke (heat-stroke) is characterized by hot dry skin, rapid breathing and a fast, weak pulse; it can be very dangerous in young children and requires immediate medical attention.

Prevention

Sunstroke can be avoided by limiting time spent in the sun and acclimatizing gradually to high temperatures.

The hottest time of the day spans from 10 a.m. to 4 p.m. It is best for a baby or young child to stay in the shade. Protect the head with a hat, dress children in light cotton clothing.

Give plenty of mineral water and dilute juices to drink to avoid dehydration. Remember that a child playing in the sun will lose a great deal of moisture through perspiration which needs to be constantly replenished.

Eating succulent fruits and vegetables will also help to preserve moisture reserves.

Practical Advice

Take a child indoors to a cool, shady room and suggest he lies down on a sofa or bed supported with cushions. Remove any clothing and sponge the body all over with cool water. Give plenty of cool drinks (not ice cold).

Homoeopathy

* Belladonna – for a hot red face and throbbing headache.
* Byronia – if symptoms are worse for movement.

Give 1 dose of the 6C potency every 2 hours for up to 4 doses.

Other Helpful Remedies

Herbal Remedies

* Lavender and Peppermint infusions can be used to sponge the body.

Aromatherapy

* Lavender or Tea Tree can be added to cool water for sponging down.

Flower Remedies

* To relieve shock give one of the emergency composites such as Rescue Remedy (Bach Flower Remedies), Five

Flower Remedy (Healing Herbs), First Aid Flower Essence (Findhorn Flower Essences) or Emergency Essence (Jan de Vries).

Give 2 drops on the tongue or in a glass of water every hour until your child seems calmer.

Doctor's Prescription

Plenty of fluids, rest in a darkened room and paracetamol for pain relief.

T

TEETHING

Teeth can start to come through any time after birth, normally beginning at around 6 months with the front incisors. Teething continues until your child has the full complement of 20 baby teeth, which may take up to 3 years. Some teeth seem to appear with no trouble at all, whereas others seem to cause great discomfort, resulting in a lot of crying and many sleepless nights.

Typical Symptoms

Inflammation and soreness of the gums, dribbling, chewing, and clingy or irritable behaviour. Other symptoms associated with teething are a snuffly nose, cough, diarrhoea, earache, restlessness and difficulty sleeping.

Practical Advice

Give baby something hard to chew on. A teething ring which can be chilled in the fridge is ideal. A stick of raw carrot is beneficial for the gums; slices of apple are good too.

Avoid commercial rusks as they often contain sugar, which causes tooth decay. Make your own home-made rusks by slow-baking hunks of bread.

Homoeopathy

* Chamomilla is the number one remedy for teething problems. Signs include over-sensitivity, with one red cheek and pain that seems intolerable. This remedy is well suited to bad-tempered children who are only quiet when carried and constantly request, then reject things. They are hot and sweaty, especially their head. Better for being uncovered, worse from 9 p.m. to midnight.

* Chamomilla is also available as drops which can be added to a bottle of milk or given diluted in cooled boiled water by the teaspoon.

* Belladonna – if cheeks are hot, red and swollen.

* Calc carb – for slow and difficult teething. The child who needs this remedy will be a slow developer, classically fat, fair and flabby.

* Pulsatilla – for the child who is clingy, weepy and whiney. Teething may be accompanied by a thick yellow nasal discharge.

Give 1 dose of the 30C potency immediately and repeat daily for up to 3 doses.

Other Helpful Remedies

Aromatherapy

* Chamomile has anti-inflammatory properties. Add 1 drop to an eggcupful of cold water and stir well. Dip a cotton wool bud in the solution and rub gently around baby's gums. Store the mixture in the fridge and use whenever it is needed.
* Make an aromatherapy oil by adding drops of Chamomile to Almond oil for massaging the cheeks and around the jawline.

Herbal Remedies

* Marshmallow Root can help to soothe inflamed or sore gums. Blend 5–10 drops of Marshmallow Root tincture with honey and massage this gently over the gums with a clean finger or cotton wool bud.
* Give teaspoons of sweetened Chamomile infusion 2 to 3 times a day.

Diet and Nutritional Therapy

* Give plenty of calcium-rich foods while the teeth are forming.

Biochemic Tissue Salts

* Calc phos or Combination R: 1 tablet every 30 minutes for up to 6 doses.

Chinese Medicine

* Work the Stomach 44 acupressure point (*see Figure 1, page 13*).

Doctor's Prescription

Teething gels containing antiseptic and analgesic ingredients may be recommended for babies over 4 months old. For distressing teething, a paracetamol solution such as *Calpol* is usually recommended to relieve pain and discomfort.

TEMPER TANTRUMS

Displays of fury and frustration which are distressing for both children and their parents. Toddlers often start to throw temper tantrums at around the age of 2 – hence the so-called 'Terrible Twos'. However, some babies may show blatant signs of anger when thwarted before they are even 1 year old.

Temper tantrums are often predictable. They tend to occur when a child cannot get his own way and resorts to rage. Sometimes they are a way of attracting attention and often begin when a sibling is born. Simply being more attentive to your child – listening to him, reading him bedtime stories – may reduce the frequency of outbursts.

Temper tantrums are also likely to occur when a child is tired, hungry or generally in a bad mood. Some natural therapists feel that food intolerances and sensitivities can spark off temper tantrums.

The occasional tantrum is to be expected, but if they happen on a regular basis you should try to do something about them.

Naturopathy

If your child throws tantrums on a daily basis there may be a dietary trigger.

* Avoid giving all processed and sugar-laden foods for at least 2 weeks to see if there is any improvement.
* Chocolate seems to spark off difficult behaviour in some children. If you suspect this to be the case, avoid

giving all products containing chocolate, such as chocolate cereals, drinks, sweets, biscuits, cakes and so forth. You might have a couple of turbulent days, but improvement should be apparent very soon.

Flower Remedies

* Heather (Bach Flower Remedies/Healing Herbs) – for those who feel needy of and greedy for the attention of others.
* Holly (Bach Flower Remedies/Healing Herbs) – for those enveloped by negative and aggressive emotions such as anger, jealousy, bitterness, envy, rage, suspicion, revenge, bad temper, contempt, selfishness and frustration.
* Mountain Devil (Australian Bush Flower Essences) – for hatred, jealousy, holding grudges and suspiciousness.
* White Carnation (Petite Fleur) – for those who are stubborn and headstrong, resulting in constant anxiety, tension and mood swings.

Give 2 drops 3 times a day until there is noticeable improvement.

Other Helpful Remedies

Herbal Remedy

* Chamomile soothes the nervous system which helps to allay temper tantrums and restores calm after the storm. Add Chamomile tincture to a glass of fruit juice or milk.

Aromatherapy

A few drops of Chamomile essential oil in the evening bath soothes the nervous system.

See also **Behavioural Problems**

THREAD WORMS

These tiny worms are particularly common in young children between the ages of 2 and 5. The eggs tend to be picked up from dirt which becomes lodged under the fingernails. When fingers or other dirty objects are put in the mouth these eggs can enter the digestive tract, where they hatch. The newly hatched eggs then travel the full length of the intestinal tract and emerge at the other end. This causes itching and scratching, which tends to perpetuate the problem.

Worms may pass from person to person so parents can also get them. The eggs can be picked up from toilet seats, other people's hands, objects handled by an infected person and even, it seems, by simply breathing in eggs circulating in the air.

The worms have a life-cycle of 2 weeks, so treatment should last at least this long to be effective.

Typical Symptoms

Itching around the anus especially in the evening, irritability, and the feeling of being slightly unwell. Worms can also be responsible for weight loss, swollen abdomen, inability to concentrate, lethargy, headaches, teeth-grinding and bedwetting.

Preventative Measures

Hygiene is the best preventative measure. Teach your child to wash his hands after going to the loo and before eating. Keep fingernails short and discourage children from putting their fingers in their mouth. If you have pets make sure they are wormed regularly. Carpets should be vacuumed every other day, particularly around and under beds. Make sure meat and fish are well-cooked. Wash all salads and vegetables carefully.

Herbal Remedies

Worms hate garlic, so adding it to dishes is one of the best natural remedies for children. If your child does not like the taste, try giving him 2 garlic capsules daily instead.

Other herbs such as Wormwood can be effective, but these should be prescribed by a professional herbalist.

Aromatherapy

* Lavender, Chamomile and Eucalyptus can help to eliminate worms and, when used regularly, keep them at bay. Add your chosen essence to a base of Almond oil and rub into the abdominal area twice a day for at least 2 weeks.

* For children over 6 years old: Niaouli can be blended with any of the other three essential oils mentioned above to enhance the potency.

* Inhaling the essences can help: add your chosen essence or blend to warm baths; 3 drops in a vaporizer can be used in your child's bedroom.

Other Helpful Remedies

Homoeopathy

* Cina – for worms in the baby who rubs and picks his nose continually, grinds teeth while asleep, has an enormous appetite or wants to eat nothing but sweet things and is generally irritable.

Diet and Nutritional Therapy

Carrots, pears and pumpkin seeds are reputed to be deterrents to worms.

Doctor's Prescription

Drugs toxic to the worms and safe for humans such as Pripsen (piperazine) or Vermox (mebendazole) will be prescribed.

THRUSH

A yeast infection which usually affects the mouth, intestines and vagina. Ordinarily this yeast, Candida albicans, lives quite harmlessly in the body. Under certain conditions it can overgrow, however, thriving in moist areas where the natural healthy bacteria have been disrupted by illness, antibiotics or oral cortico-steroids, or anything which compromises the immune system. Candida can also flourish when the natural acidity of the vagina becomes more alkaline, generally as a result of hormonal upheavals, but also the over-use of bubble baths and soap. When Candida gets out of control it gives rise to various symptoms.

Typical Symptoms

White patches or coating on the tongue; a cottage cheese-like discharge in the vagina giving rise to inflammation, itching and stinging. May be accompanied by feelings of nausea, irritability, headache, abdominal bloating and overwhelming cravings for sweet, sugary foods.

In babies, thrush commonly occurs as white curd-like spots on the tongue and inside the cheeks. It is more prevalent in babies whose mothers also have thrush or have recently taken antibiotics. If not treated at an early stage it can travel to their bottom, causing a form of nappy rash which looks like tiny red spots.

Suspect thrush if the rash starts around the anus and spreads outwards and up towards the navel.

If baby is breastfeeding, the thrush may spread to mother's nipples, making them particularly sore. After each feed it is a good idea to wash the nipples with warm water to prevent infection.

Diet and Nutritional Therapy

Candida, like all yeasts, thrives on sugar. Avoid giving sweet foods including fruit (especially dried fruits), fruit juices (unless diluted 50:50 with water) and honey.

Fermented (yeast-containing) foods and fungi may exacerbate thrush, so avoid foods such as bread, yeast extract (*Marmite*), vinegar, mushrooms, smoked fish, sausages, soy sauce and cheese to see if symptoms start to clear.

Give plenty of natural 'live' yoghurt (with *Lactobacillus acidophilus* culture) – at least a carton a day – the acidophilus bacteria help to keep the yeast in check. A supplement of acidophilus and bifidus bacteria (available from healthfood stores) will help to replenish healthy bacteria and ward off thrush. Give one capsule (half a teaspoon of powder) twice daily for 1 month.

Olive oil inhibits the growth of yeast and should be included in the diet as often as possible – at least 1 tablespoon a day.

Whey, a by-product of cheese-making, contains lactic acid which helps to create conditions that are hostile to Candida. It can be used as a mouthwash; taken internally it will help restore the correct pH balance in the gut.

Herbal Remedies

* Aloe Vera juice can help to combat thrush and, used neat, makes a good mouthwash. It can also be given as a drink: 10 ml 2 to 3 times a day on its own or mixed with vegetable juice.
* Caprylic acid, an extract of coconuts, has powerful anti-fungal properties. Children over 2 years old can be given 3 capsules a day at mealtimes.
* Garlic is a potent anti-fungal agent. Include plenty of fresh garlic in cooking, or give 2 capsules 3 times a day.

Other Helpful Remedies

Homoeopathy

- * Try Borax at the first sign of symptoms.
- * Kali mur – for breastfeeding babies whose tongue and gums are coated white and whose symptoms are worse for feeding and touch. Also for genital thrush with burning, itchy discharge. Try Sepia if the thrush has infected mother's nipples too.

Give 1 dose of the 30C potency daily for up to 3 doses.

Aromatherapy

- * Tea Tree has potent anti-fungal properties and can be used for babies over 6 months old. Add this essence to the bath.
- * For children over 3 years old: Make a mouthwash using 2 drops of Tea Tree in 50 ml of tepid (previously boiled) water.

Doctor's Prescription

Anti-fungal Nystatin suspension is prescribed for mouth infections; anti-fungal creams such as Canesten (clotrimazole) for nappy rash or vaginal thrush.

Seek help if the thrush does not respond to home treatment and your baby or child is obviously miserable; if your nipples become infected or if pus forms.

Compare **Nappy Rash, Rashes**

TONSILLITIS

Inflammation and swelling of the tonsils, a condition that most commonly occurs in children. The tonsils are a first line of defence against all bacteria and viruses, and frequently flare up in response to any infection.

Typical Symptoms

Sore throat, difficulty and pain when swallowing, white or red deposits on the tonsils, fever and sometimes a congested chest and nose. The sufferer feels unwell and may have a headache, neck ache, tummy ache and be susceptible to earache.

Diet and Nutritional Therapy

Follow the same guidelines given for a **Sore Throat**.

Herbal Remedies

* Red Sage infusion makes an effective gargle for soothing inflammation. Encourage your child to gargle 3 times a day, more frequently if possible.
* An infusion of Marshmallow leaves and flowers sweetened with honey will soothe the throat.
* Rose and Geranium syrups are soothing remedies for tonsillitis. Prepare during the summer for use during the colder months. You will need:

   Flowers or petals to fill a pint/600-ml jar.

   20 fl oz/600 ml of water

   3 drops of Rose or Geranium essential oil

   2.2 lb/1 kg of sugar

   Add freshly picked flowers to the water and bring to the boil. Turn down the heat and simmer for 10 minutes. Leave to cool for a further 10 minutes, strain and top up the water level to 600 ml. Add the sugar to the water and heat, stirring until the mixture thickens. Add the essential oils and a few more flowers to the syrup. Pour into jars and store in the refrigerator. Give 1 teaspoon 3 times a day.

Elderflower Syrup (*see page 31*) is another option.

Children's Immunity Formula (*see page 32*) can help the body to fight off the infection: 10 drops in 6 fl oz/180 ml water 3 times a day until recovery is complete.

Homoeopathy

If your child suffers recurrent bouts of tonsillitis consult a professional homoeopath who can prescribe a constitutional remedy for strengthening the body's resistance.

Various remedies will help to relieve the acute symptoms:

* Aconite – for swollen tonsils, burning throat which comes on suddenly and is made worse by cold wind. Everything will taste bitter to the sufferer who needs this remedy.
* Gelsemium – for pain in the neck and ears, pain on swallowing, flu-like aching and weakness.
* Hepar sulph – for stitching pain (like swallowing a splinter) which extends to the ears when swallowing, pus-filled lesions on the tonsils, hypersensitivity to everything including touch and noise.
* You could also try Apis mel or Merc sol for pain on the left side, Belladonna for pain on the right side.

Give the 6C potency, 1 dose every hour for up to 4 doses. Repeat as necessary.

Other Helpful Remedies

Aromatherapy

* Lemon and Ginger can be used for a mouthwash. Add

4 drops of either essence to 50 ml of tepid (previously boiled) water.

* For children over 6 years old: You can use a mixture of both essences (2 drops of each).
* Swish around the mouth 3 times a day.
* Sprinkle 4 drops of your chosen oil on a warm compress and apply to the throat area twice a day, or make up a massage oil and rub into the neck and jaw area.

Chinese Medicine

* Add 10 drops of Chinese dandelion tincture to 1 cup/240 ml of tepid (previously boiled) water and use as a gargle.
* Work the Large Intestine 4 and Stomach 44 acupressure points (*see Figure 1, page 13*).

Biochemic Tissue Salts

* Kali mur: 2 tablets every 2 hours for up to 6 doses, then 3 times daily.

Doctor's Prescription

Gargling with salt water may be recommended to combat infection and soothe the tonsils, together with a paracetamol solution to relieve pain and reduce fever, and possibly antibiotics to combat the infection.

TRAVEL SICKNESS

The feeling of nausea and sickness that accompanies travelling is a common complaint in children of all ages. While car journeys often have a soporific effect on babies, some babies and young children hate them, which suggests they may also suffer from travel sickness. If your baby is sick or cries when put in the car, this could be the reason.

Travel sickness is a result of motion disturbing the balance mechanism within the inner ear. Any form of journey, whether by car, train, plane or boat, may bring on travel sickness. The nervous anticipation of travelling can even bring on symptoms.

Typical Symptoms

Nausea, sickness, dizziness, headache, sweating, pallor and fatigue.

Practical Advice

In the car:
* Whenever possible a child will fare better when sitting in the front seat or where he can see the road ahead.
* Always keep a window slightly open to ensure there is plenty of fresh air.
* Never smoke in the car.
* Pack plenty of toys to keep your baby or child busy and less aware of the journey, but discourage reading or playing games which require focusing on moving stationary objects inside the car.

On a boat:
* It is best to be on deck where the horizon can be seen. Enclosed spaces 'down below' increase feelings of nausea.
* Stay around the mid-line of the boat, as this part oscillates less than the sides.

On a train:
* Try to ensure that your child is facing the direction in which the train is moving.

On a plane:
* Try to keep your child occupied, as advised in the section on car travel, above.

Diet and Nutritional Therapy

* Give a light meal before any journey, such as a bowl of cereal, a piece of lightly buttered toast or sandwich. Any sweet or fatty foods should be avoided.
* Apples, pears, raw carrots or grapes make ideal snacks during journeys – and good substitutes for crisps, sweets, ice cream and chocolate.
* Give bottled spring water and dilute fruit juices to quench thirst.

Herbal Remedies

* Ginger is one of the best natural remedies for travel sickness. Scientific studies suggest it is as effective as orthodox medicines for quelling feelings of nausea and sickness. Give pieces of crystallized ginger to chew, and make ginger biscuits with plenty of added stem ginger for the journey. If your child does not like the taste you could try giving him ginger tablets to swallow.
* Peppermint will help to settle the stomach and relieve feelings of nausea. Give Peppermint tablets to suck and sprinkle a few drops of Peppermint oil onto a tissue to inhale.

Other Helpful Remedies

Chinese Medicine

Working the Pericardium 6 or *Nei Kuan* acupressure point (*see Figure 1, page 13*) can work wonders for preventing and relieving travel sickness. Several research studies have proven the efficacy of holding this point. In one Italian study, Seabands (armbands with a rubber button that massages the point) were used on children known to suffer from violent travel sickness. For **88.7 per** cent the results were excellent; for the remainder, nausea was much reduced. A child can also be taught how to find and massage this point as a self-help measure.

Homoeopathy

* Petroleum is one of the main travel-sickness remedies – for nausea, dizziness and vomiting; symptoms worse for fresh air and morning travel.
* Tabacum – for nausea that is more acute when travelling by boat and vomiting is worse when travelling by car or train. Better for fresh air. Worse for stuffy atmosphere, movement and cigarette smoke.
* You could also try Ipecac for nausea felt in the head, without vomiting, or Cocculus for vomiting with profuse salivation and a complete aversion to the smell of food.

Give 1 dose of the 6C potency hourly as soon as symptoms begin.

Aromatherapy

* For babies: Fennel and Dill can ease symptoms when inhaled. Make an aromatherapy oil and massage into the chest, or sprinkle a few drops on a tissue and tuck into the seat straps in the car.
* For children over 1 year old: You can also use Peppermint.

Reflexology

A workout can help to calm a child before a journey. If there is too little time, a few presses to the solar plexus reflex area on the hand or foot will be beneficial (*see Figure 2, page 53*). Showing your child how to do this will help to keep him occupied, too.

Doctor's Prescription

Medication is rarely recommended as children are very sensitive to drugs used to prevent sickness and can suffer side-effects. Phenergan may be helpful.

Compare **Sickness and Nausea**

V

VACCINATIONS

The purpose of vaccination (or immunization) is to induce immunity as a protective measure against certain infectious illnesses. It involves injecting or administering by mouth slightly modified organisms which stimulate the body's production of antibodies, so that if the actual virus or bacterium is encountered the immune system can recognize and deal with it more efficiently.

The childhood immunization timetable begins shortly after birth, normally at 2 months of age, with vaccinations against Diphtheria, Whooping Cough, Tetanus, Polio and Hib (bacterial meningitis).

Between 12 and 15 months of age babies are given the Measles, Mumps and Rubella (MMR) vaccination.

At around 3–5 years vaccination against Diphtheria, Tetanus and Polio is repeated.

Vaccination is not compulsory and the decision of whether or not to have your child immunized against all or any of these diseases is not an easy one to make. Most natural healthcare practitioners, in particular naturopaths, homoeopaths and osteopaths, question the benefits of vaccination because they have seen formerly healthy children become chronically ill after being given certain vaccines. It is thought that vaccination may make excessive demands on the immature defences of young infants which, in the long term, may undermine health. Known and suspected side-effects of vaccination include increased allergies, a worsening of asthma or eczema, recurrent ear infections, fatigue states and learning disabilities. Both the measles and rubella immunizations have been linked to rheumatoid arthritis in young people and, more recently, the MMR vaccine has been associated with the increased incidence of Crohn's disease, a debilitating disorder of the bowel.

Natural therapists maintain that a strong immune system offers the best form of defence against any kind of infection, and this results from breastfeeding, a nutrient-rich diet and healthy lifestyle including natural treatment for minor ailments. A child cared for in this way should be less vulnerable to childhood diseases and, if they occur, symptoms will be mild and recovery swift.

The illnesses themselves, on the other hand, can carry risks and it may be irresponsible not to immunize a child against potentially lethal infections such as Tetanus, Polio and Diphtheria.

It is beyond the scope of this book to go into the issue of vaccination in any depth. Before making a choice one way or another it is a parent's responsibility to weigh up all the pros and cons. Recommended reading includes *Vaccination and Immunization: What Does Your Child Need?* by Anne Charlish (Thorsons) and the *What Doctors Don't Tell You Vaccination Handbook* (Wallace Press).

Alternatives to Vaccination

Homoeopathy

If you decide against immunization, professional homoeopathic treatment should be given to boost your child's natural immunity.

In addition, homoeopathy offers a range of remedies known as 'nosodes' which can be given as preventative measures when there is an outbreak or epidemic of certain childhood illnesses. These can be extremely effective, but should only be used following consultation with a qualified homoeopath.

Homoeopathic Prophylactics

Chicken pox	Varicella 30
Diphtheria	Diphtherium 30
German measles	Rubella 30
Hib	Hib 30
Measles	Moribillinum 30
Mumps	Parotidinum 30
Polio	Polio 30
Whooping Cough	Pertussin 30

If your child does contract any of these infections, homoeopathic remedies may help to alleviate the intensity of the illness and reduce the likelihood of complications.

Diet and Nutritional Therapy

Immunity can be boosted with a varied wholefood diet rich in vitamins A, C and E and the mineral zinc, nutrients known to play a vital role in ensuring that the immune system functions efficiently.

Medical research suggests that giving vitamin A to children with severe measles lessens the risk of complications.

The best source of vitamin A is beta carotene, which abounds in green- and orange-coloured fruits and vegetables. It is converted into vitamin A in the body.

Recommended Daily Doses of Beta Carotene:

1–5 years old	2,500 international units (iu)
5–12 years old	5,000 iu

Natural Antidotes to Vaccination

If you decide to have your child vaccinated, there are ways to minimize any adverse effects:

Delay vaccination if your child is suffering from a cold or seems below par.

Prepare your baby or child for vaccination with nourishing meals and freshly squeezed fruit and vegetable juices. A lack of many nutrients, particularly vitamins B_6 and B_5, impairs the body's ability to produce antibodies and so decreases the effectiveness of various vaccines.

Nutritional Therapy

Vitamin C helps to strengthen the immune response and neutralize the viral and bacterial toxins. Give babies 250 mg, added to fresh fruit juice, before and directly after the vaccination. Breastfed babies benefit if mother takes 1 g of vitamin C. Children over 3 years old can be given 500 mg vitamin C before and after vaccination.

Flower Remedies

* Rescue Remedy (Bach Flower Remedies/Healing Herbs) or First Aid Remedy (Findhorn Flower Essences) – to relieve the shock. Give 2 drops before vaccination and again immediately afterwards. Repeat the dosage every 2 hours until your child seems calmer, then give 3 times daily for the next 2 to 3 days.

Homoeopathy

Once your child has been immunized:

* Aconite – for shock.
* Arnica – for bruising at the site of the injection.
* Staphysagria – for anger, betrayal, hurt and resentment.
* Stramonium – if your child suffers from nightmares afterward immunization.

Give the 6C potency, 1 dose immediately and every 2 hours for up to 4 doses.

A professional homoeopath can prescribe remedies to help your child regain his former vitality if you suspect that his health has suffered as a result of vaccination.

Doctor's Prescription

Most doctors are in favour of the full immunization programme as a preventative measure against disease. They are of the opinion that serious illness as a direct consequence of immunization is extremely rare, and that any risks outweigh those of contracting the disease itself. Measles, for example, can have severe and even fatal consequences for a few children. Common reactions to inoculations include a mild viral type of illness with a temperature with swelling and redness at the injection site, all of which soon pass.

See also **Childhood Diseases**

VERRUCAS *See* **Warts and Verrucas**

VOMITING *See* **Sickness and Nausea**

W

WARTS AND VERRUCAS

Warts and verrucas are harmless yet contagious growths which are spread by a virus. Warts look like little lumps and are commonly found on the hands and fingers, although they can grow anywhere. Verrucas are warts on the feet that grow upwards into the fleshy part of the foot, which means they can be quite painful.

Warts seldom appear before the age of 2, and most go away by themselves without any therapy other than patience. Warts can take anything from 6 months to 3 years to disappear of their own accord. Intriguingly, children with eczema (overactive skin immunity) have fewer warts than other children.

A folk remedy has it that keeping warts in the dark will speed their disappearance. It seems to prompt the immune system into attacking the wart and many clear in 6 weeks with this simple cover-up treatment. Cover with a plaster for a week, remove the plaster, wash the area and let it dry, then repeat the procedure.

Natural remedies may help warts to clear faster than if left to live out their natural life span, but don't expect miracles.

Homoeopathy

Homoeopaths regard warts and verrucas as part of an overall symptom picture which can be cured with a constitutional treatment. They feel that suppressing warts with, for example, topical acids can lead to the development of more serious complaints.

Remedies to try at home are:

* Ant crud – for flat horny warts on the hands and soles of the feet.
* Causticum – for large jagged warts on the face, fingertips or eyelids which bleed easily.
* Nit ac – for cauliflower-like warts that are itchy and bleed when washed.

Give 1 dose of the 30C potency weekly.

Thuja tincture can be applied twice a day. Keep the wart covered between applications.

Other Helpful Remedies

Aromatherapy

* Lemon is one of the best essences for treating warts and verrucas. Apply 2 drops to a teaspoon of lemon juice. Dip a cotton wool bud into the solution and apply directly, to the infected area only, twice a day.
* For children over 7 years old: Cypress can be used in combination with Lemon. Put 10 drops of Lemon and 5 drops of Cypress in a dessertspoon of cider vinegar. Pour into a clean bottle, shake well and use this mixture as above.

Herbal Remedy

* Rubbing raw garlic onto a wart is said to help remove it. Adding plenty of fresh garlic to the diet may also help.

Professional Therapy

Deep Relaxation/Hypnosis

This therapy may be very effective at getting rid of warts. In one study, 10 patients with warts on both sides of the body were told, under hypnosis, that the warts would disappear from just one side. In 9 out of the 10 patients this is just what happened. Children have particularly good imaginations, and suggesting ways of getting the warts to disappear – such as rubbing them with a banana skin and burying it in the garden, just might do the trick!

Doctor's Prescription

If verrucas and warts do not hurt it is best to leave them, as they eventually disappear. If troublesome they can be killed by freezing with liquid nitrogen or caustic ointment.

WHOOPING COUGH (PERTUSSIS)

A serious infectious disease affecting the respiratory system. Whooping cough, or pertussis, commonly affects infants and young children, with around half the cases occurring before the age of 2. Babies receive no passive immunity from their mother. This means they are susceptible to the infection from birth, which is when whooping cough is most dangerous. In general, the younger the child, the greater the risks.

A characteristic feature is very severe bouts of coughing which may hang on for several weeks. The symptoms are caused by a bacterium which infects the lungs and causes the airways to become clogged with a thick layer of mucus. One bout of coughing may follow another, which is exhausting and can make it very difficult for the child to breathe.

In young babies there is a danger of not being able to breathe properly after a coughing fit; feeding is also a struggle. Whooping cough is a long and tiring infection for both child and parent, as it can last from 3 weeks to 4 months.

Typical Symptoms

First signs are a slight fever, runny nose, mild, dry cough, slight temperature and pink, watery eyes; resembles a cold. After a few days symptoms get worse. As the mucus thickens, coughing fits follow with the characteristic 'whoop' as air is drawn in. There may also be nosebleeds and vomiting. The severe coughing phase may last from 2 to 10 weeks. The illness brings exhaustion and sometimes permanent lung damage.

Practical Advice

Always consult your doctor and obtain professional assistance in treating a child with whooping cough.

Treatment is not simple, but with special care and perseverance the symptoms can be managed.

Keep your child away from other children for at least 12 weeks. Even an immunized child can catch a mild form of this disease and so become infectious, even though his symptoms resemble those of a cold or cough.

Follow the general guidelines for **Childhood Diseases**; *see also* **Infections**.

Diet and Nutritional Therapy

* Avoid giving dairy products, which can encourage the formation of excess mucus.

* As well as giving plenty of drinks, offer soothing home-made sorbets made from diluted natural fruit juices to suck.
* Make nourishing soups from liquidized vegetables so they are easy to swallow. Onions, turnips, watercress, cabbage and garlic are beneficial for the chest and respiratory system. Try to give your child some of this soup every day.

Homoeopathy

* Drosera is the number one remedy for whooping cough – for a violent, spasmodic cough that leads to gagging/vomiting or nosebleed. The sufferer will feel the sensation of a feather in the throat and be restless, emotionally stubborn or suspicious. All symptoms improve after midnight and are better for sitting up, open air; worse for lying down, talking, warmth.
* Belladonna – for fever with hot head/headache, glassy eyes and barking cough.

Other Helpful Remedies

Aromatherapy

* For babies and children under 5 years old: use Lavender only. Place 2 drops of the essential oil on a tissue and place near your child so he can inhale it. Lavender can also be added to the bath.
* For children over 5 years old: use a blend of Lavender, Niaouli and Hyssop. Sprinkle 1 drop of each on a tissue tucked into the pillow for inhaling or in a vaporizer in your child's room. One drop of each can also be added to the bath.

Naturopathy

* Place bowls of steaming water in your child's room at night (with added essential oils; *see above*) to keep the atmosphere as humid as possible.
* Open the windows to ensure there is plenty of fresh air.

Professional Therapies

Herbal Remedies

Various herbs, such as Coltsfoot, Elecampane, Aniseed and Liquorice can be helpful but should always be prescribed by a qualified herbalist for this serious condition.

Homoeopathy

It is advisable to consult a professional homoeopath to help with home prescribing and managing this illness. As a preventative measure against whooping cough, Pertussin 30C can be given.

Doctor's Prescription

Routine vaccination against whooping cough (pertussis) is recommended during the first year of life. Most babies are given a combination of whooping cough, diphtheria and tetanus (DPT) together with Hib at 2, 3 and 4 months of age.

If the illness is recognized early, antibiotics may be given as a safeguard against complications such as chest infections.

Seek emergency help if a child becomes blue or vomits continuously after a coughing fit.

Addresses

AROMATHERAPY

Academy of Aromatherapy and Massage
50 Cow Wynd
Falkirk
Sterlingshire FK1 1OU

International Federation of Aromatherapists
Stamford House
2–4 Chiswick High Road
London W4 1TH

International Society of Professional Aromatherapists
ISPA House
82 Ashby Road
Hinckley
Leics PE10 1SN

ESSENTIAL OILS AND AROMATHERAPY PREPARATIONS

Neal's Yard Remedies
2 Neal's Yard
Covent Garden
London WC2
 and
5 Golden Cross
Cornmarket Street
Oxford OX1 3EU

Tisserand Institute
65 Church Road
Hove
East Sussex BN3 2BD

ACUPRESSURE

The Shen Tao Foundation
Middle Piccadilly Natural Healing Centre
Holwell
Sherbourne
Dorset DT9 5LW

CHINESE HERBAL REMEDIES

Home-made preparations and tinctures available directly from:
Katharine Jackson
72 Waterford Road
London SW6 2DR

Neal's Yard Remedies
See address above

Register of Chinese Herbal Medicine
PO Box 400
Wembley
Middlesex HA9 9NZ

DIET AND NUTRITIONAL THERAPY

British Nutrition Foundation
High Holborn House
52–54 High Holborn
London WC1 6RQ

Institute for Optimum Nutrition
13 Blades Court
Deodor Road
London SW15 2NU

FLOWER REMEDIES

International Federation for Vibrational Medicine
Middle Piccadilly Healing Centre
Holwell
Dorset

Can provide a list of fully qualified flower remedy practitioners

Bach Flower Remedies
Dr Edward Bach Centre
Mount Vernon
Sotwell
Wallingford
Oxon OX10 OPZ

Bush Flower Essences of Australia
8a Oaks Avenue
Dee Why
New South Wales
2099
Australia

Findhorn Flower Essences
Mercury
Findhorn Bay
Forres
Morayshire IV36 OTY

Flower Essence Society
PO Box 459
Nevada City
CA 95959,
USA

Healing Herbs – The Flower Remedy Programme
PO Box 65
Hereford HR2 OUW

International Flower Essence Repertoire
The Working Tree
Millard
Liphook
Hampshire GU30 7JS

Can supply flower essences from around the world

Laboratoire Deva Elixirs Floreaux
BP 3 – 38880 Autrans, France

Living Essences of Australia
Box 355 Scarborough, Perth
West Australia
6019

Pacific Essences
PO Box 8317
Victoria
British Columbia
V8W 3R9
Canada

Petite Fleur Essences Inc.
8524 Whispering Creek Trail
Fort Worth
TX 76134,
USA

The Hale Clinic
7 Park Crescent
London W1N 3HE

The shop carries a selection of key essences from around the world including Jan de Vries Emergency Essence

HERBALISM

National Institute of Medical Herbalists
41 Hatherley Road
Winchester
Hants

Have a register of professional herbalists

HERBAL REMEDIES

Bioforce(UK) Ltd
Dundonald KA2 9BE

G Baldwin and Co
171 Walworth Road
London SE17 1RW

Gerard House Ltd
836 Christchurch Road
Bournemouth BH7 6BZ

Hambleden Herbs
Court Farm
Milverton
Taunton
Somerset TA4 1NF

Suppliers of fresh and dried organic herbs

Herbs Hands Healing
2 Bridge Farm Cottages
Station Road
Pulham Market IP21 4TF

Can supply ready-made Little Ones' Cough Syrup and Happy Child Formula

Neal's Yard Remedies
See address above

Potter's (Herbal Suppliers) Ltd
Douglas Words
Leyland Mill Lane
Wigan
Lancs WN1 2BS

Sunflower Vital Health Initiative
17 Bristol Road
Ilkeston
Derbyshire DE7 5HD

Can provide ready-made herbal remedies such as Children's Stress, Children's Immunity, Immune Balance and Happy Child formulas

Weleda (UK) Ltd
Heanor Road
Ilkeston
Derbyshire DE7 8DR

HOMOEOPATHY

British Homoeopathic Association
27A Devonshire Street
London W1N 1RJ

Send SAE for list of practitioners

Society of Homoeopaths
2 Artizan Road
Northampton NN1 4HU

Send SAE for register of professional homoeopaths

HOMOEOPATHIC REMEDIES

Ainsworths Homoeopathic Pharmacy
38 New Cavendish Street
London W1M 7LH

Helios Homoeopathic Pharmacy
97 Camden Road
Tunbridge Wells
Kent TN1 1QP

Have a range of special kits with small refillable bottles of key remedies

Neal's Yard Remedies
See address above

Nelsons Homoeopathic Preparations
available from Boots the Chemist and most healthfood stores

Weleda (UK) Ltd
See address above

HYDROTHERAPY

British Naturopathic and Osteopathic Association
See address below

UK College of Hydrotherapy
515 Hagley Road
Birmingham B66 4AX

MASSAGE

London College of Massage
5 Newman Passage
London W1P 3PF

NATUROPATHY

British Naturopathic and Osteopathic Association
Frazer House
6 Netherhall Gardens
London NW3 5RR

A list of qualified naturopaths can be obtained from the General Council and Register or Naturopaths (GCRN) at this address:

General Council and Register of Naturopaths
Goswell House
2 Goswell Road
Somerset BA16 OJG

OSTEOPATHY

General Register and Council of Osteopaths
56 London Street
Reading
Berkshire RG1 4SQ

Osteopathic Centre for Children
4 Harcourt House
19a Cavendish Square
London W1M 9AD

REFLEXOLOGY

Association of Reflexologists
27 Old Gloucester Street
London WC1N 3XX

British School of Reflexology and Holistic Association of Reflexologists
92 Sheering Road
Old Harlow
Essex CM17 OJW

International Federation of Reflexologists
76–78 Edridge Road
Croydon
Surrey CR10 1EF

International Institute of Reflexology
15 Hartfield Close
Tonbridge
Kent

RELAXATION

Association of Stress Therapists
5 Springfied Road
Palm Bay
Cliftonville
Kent CT9 3EA

References and Further Reading

Belinda Barnes and Irene Colquhoun, *The Hyperactive Child* (HarperCollins, 1984)

Miranda Castro, *Homoeopathy for Mother and Baby* (Macmillan, 1992)

Leon Chaitow, *Water Therapy* (Thorsons, 1994)

Anne Charlish, *Vaccination and Immunization: What does your child need* (Thorsons, 1996)

Susan Curtis, Rony Fraser and Irene Kohler, *Neal's Yard Natural Remedies* (Arkana Penguin, 1988)

Dr Stephen Davies and Dr Alan Stewart, *Nutritional Medicine* (Pan Books, 1987)

Adelle Davis, *Let's Have Healthy Children* (Unwin Paperbacks, 1984)

Nalda Gosling, *Successful Herbal Remedies* (Thorsons, 1985)

Dr David Haslam, *Sleepless Children* (Piatkus, 1992)

Clare G. Harvey and Amanda Cochrane, *The Encyclopaedia of Flower Remedies* (Thorsons, 1995)

Carol Hunter, *The Best Healthy Baby Cookbook* (HarperCollins, 1985, 1990)

Joseph M. Kadans, *The Encyclopaedia of Medicinal Foods* (Thorsons, 1982)

References and Further Reading

Leslie Kenton, *Nature's Child* (Ebury Press, 1993)

Julian Kenyon, *Acupressure Techniques* (Thorsons, 1987)

Kevin and Barbara Kunz, *Reflexology for Children* (Thorsons, 1996)

Richard Lucas, *Secrets of the Chinese Herbalists* (NY: Parker Publishing Company, 1987)

Shirley Price and Penny Parr, *Aromatherapy for Babies and Children* (Thorsons, 1996)

Daniele Ryman, *The Aromatherapy Handbook* (Century Publishing, 1984)

Daniele Ryman, *Aromatherapy in Your Diet* (Piatkus, 1996)

Ellyn Satter, *Child of Mine – Feeding with Love and Good Sense* (CA: Bull Publishing Company, 1991)

Angela Smyth, *Gentle Medicine: Thorsons Concise Encyclopaedia of Natural Health* (Thorsons, 1994)

The Reader's Digest Association Ltd, *Reader's Digest Family Guide to Alternative Medicine* (The Reader's Digest Association Ltd, 1991)

Hetty Van de Rijt and Frans Plooij, *Why They Cry* (Thorsons, 1996)

The Wallace Press, *The What Doctors Don't Tell You Vaccination Handbook* (The Wallace Press, 1989 to 1996)

Caroline Wheater, *Juicing for Health* (Thorsons, 1993)

Valerie Ann Worwood, *The Fragrant Pharmacy* (Macmillan, 1990)

Index

accidents 60–62
aches 62–4
aconite 58
acupressure 11–13
allergies 64–6, 157–60
almond milk 159
Aloe vera juice/gel 58
animal bites 86
anxiety 67–70
appetite problems 150–52
arnica 58
aromatherapy 2–7, 57
asthma 70–77
athlete's foot 77–9

Bach flower remedies 24–7
bedwetting 80–83
behaviour problems 83–6
bifidophilus supplements 57, 139, 260
biochemic tissue salts 8–10
bites 86–9
blood sugar 202
breastmilk 21–2, 180–81
bronchiolitis 89–91
bronchitis 89–91
bruises 91–3
burns 93–5

calendula cream 37, 58
Candida albicans 259–61
chamomilla drops 58
chicken pox 96–8, 99–102
Chinese herbal remedies 14–16
Chinese medicine 10–16
coeliac disease 102–4
colds 104–8
colic 108–12
conjunctivitis 113–15
constipation 115–17
cough syrups 31
coughs 118–21
cradle cap 121–3
cranial osteopathy 51
croup 123–5
crying 125–9
cuts 129–30
cystitis 131–4

depression 135–7
diarrhoea 138–41
diet 16–24, 48, 57
drawing ointment 31

ear infections 142–5
earache 142–5
eating problems 150–52
Echinacea tincture 57

Index

eczema 145–9
elderflower syrup 31
Emergency Essence 57
enuresis 80–83
essential oils 3–7, 57

fears 216–18
feeding problems 150–52
Feingold diet 173–4
fever 152–7
First Aid Essence 57
first aid kit 57–8
Five Flower Remedy 57
flower remedies 24–7, 57
flu 185–7
food 16–24, 150–52
food allergies 157–60

garlic capsules 57
German measles 99–102, 225–7
ginger, crystallized 58
glass, drawing ointment 31
gluten sensitivity 102–4

happy child formula 33
hay fever 161–6
headaches 166–9
headlice 195–7
heat rashes 222–3
herbal medicine 14–16, 27–33, 57–8
hiccups 170
hives 171–2
homoeopathy 33–8, 58
hydrotherapy 39–41
hyperactivity 172–6

Hypercal 37–8
hypericum cream 37–8, 58
immune balance formula 32
immune system 180–81
immunity formula 32
immunization 269–73
impetigo 177–9
infections 179–84
infectious illnesses 99–102
influenza 185–7
injuries 60–62
insect bites and stings 86–9
insomnia 236–40
iron deficiency 18
irritability 187–9

jaundice 190–91
juices 20, 48

lactose intolerance 192–3
laryngitis 193–5
lice 195–7

massage 42–6
measles 99–102, 198–201
meditation 57
mental growth spurts 125–6
milk, lactose intolerance 157, 159, 192–3
minerals 23–4, 57
moodiness 202–3
mouth ulcers 203–5
mumps 99–102, 205–8
nappy rash 209–12
naturopathy 47–9
nausea 230–34

nettle rash 171–2
night terrors 212–14
nightmares 212–14
nits 195–7
nosebleeds 214–15
nutritional therapy 16–24, 57

organic food 20–21
osteopathy 49–51

pains 62–4
pertussis 99–102, 276–9
phobias 216–18
pink eye 113–15
psoriasis 218–21

rashes 101–2, 222–3
reflexology 51–4
reform diet 48
relaxation 55–7
Rescue Remedy 57
rest 55–7
rhinitis 161–6
ringworm 223–5
rubella 99–102, 225–7

scalds 93–5
scratches 129–30
separation anxiety 67–8
shock 228–30
sickness 230–34
sinusitis 234–5
sleep 55
  problems 236–40
Slippery Elm powder 58
sore throat 242–4

splinters, drawing ointment 31
spotty illnesses, recipe 101–2
stings 86–9
stomach ache 244–7
  see also colic
stress formula 32
sunburn 247–9
sunstroke 249–51

teething 153, 252–5
temper tantrums 255–6
temperature, high 152–7
thermometer, use 153
thorns, drawing ointment 31
thread worms 257–9
throat, sore 242–4
thrush 259–61
tissue salts 8–10
tonsillitis 261–4
travel sickness 264–8
travelling, and food 138–9

urtica urens cream 37
urticaria 171–2

vaccinations 269–73
verrucas 274–6
vitamins 23, 57
vomiting 230–34

warts 274–6
water, drinking 40–41
water therapy 39–41
whooping cough 99–102, 276–9
worms 257–9

zinc deficiency 18